MY BODY, MY SELF

FOR BOYS

OTHER BOOKS BY LYNDA MADARAS

Ready, Set, Grow!
A *"WHAT'S HAPPENING TO MY BODY?"* BOOK FOR YOUNGER GIRLS

My Feelings, My Self for Girls
AND AREA MADARAS

The "What's Happening to My Body?" Book for Girls
WITH AREA MADARAS

The "What's Happening to My Body?" Book for Boys
WITH AREA MADARAS

My Body, My Self for Girls
AND AREA MADARAS

*Lynda Madaras Talks to Teens About AIDS: An Essential Guide
for Parents, Teachers, and Young People*

Womancare: A Gynecological Guide to Your Body
WITH JANE PATTERSON, M.D.

Woman Doctor: The Education of Jane Patterson, M.D.
WITH JANE PATTERSON, M.D.

Great Expectations
WITH LEIGH ADAMS

The Alphabet Connection
WITH PAM PALEWICZ-ROUSSEAU

Child's Play

MY BODY, MY SELF

FOR BOYS

LYNDA MADARAS
AND AREA MADARAS

WM

WILLIAM MORROW

An Imprint of HarperCollins*Publishers*

FOR OUR FATHERS

HarperCollins books may be purchased for educational, business, or sales promotional use. For information please write: Special Markets Department, HarperCollins Publishers, 10 East 53rd Street, New York, NY 10022.

FIRST WILLIAM MORROW PAPERBACK EDITION PUBLISHED 2012.

Library of Congress Cataloging-in-Publication Data

Madaras, Lynda.

  My body, my self for boys / Lynda Madaras and Area Madaras.—2nd rev. ed.

    p. cm.

  Includes bibliographical references and index.

  ISBN 978-1-55704-767-0 (pbk.)   1. Teenage boys—Growth—Juvenile literature.
2. Teenage boys—Physiology—Juvenile literature. 3. Puberty—Juvenile literature. 4. Sex instruction for boys—Juvenile literature. 1. Madaras, Area. II. Title.

RJ143.M327 2007
613.9'53—dc22

                                                                                                2007009864

Book design by Kris Tobiassen
All drawings by Simon Sullivan except for pages i, 9, 10, 13, 49, 63, 66, 80, 81, 91, 109, 111, and 113 by Artzooks Creative Group

        14   15   16   RRD   9   8   7   6   5

CONTENTS

ACKNOWLEDGMENTS

We'd like to thank all the men and boys who made this book possible by sharing their feelings and experiences with us. Thanks to Andrew F., Chico F., Michael F., Moshe F., Victor F., Jonathan K., Michael L., Andy M., George M., John O., Warren O., Tracy R., Larry S., Everett T., Big Al V., Bill V., the boys in our classes and workshops, and the many boys and men who have written to us over the years.

PREFACE

Hi, we're Lynda and Area Madaras.

We're the mother-and-daughter team who put this book together (with a lot of help from our friends). We've been writing books and teaching classes on puberty and sexuality for years. We have also written another book called *The "What's Happening to My Body?" Book for Boys* that explains the physical and emotional changes a boy goes through during his preteen and teen years, as his body changes from a child's into a man's body. This time of change is known as puberty, and the book explains how and why puberty happens and answers the many questions that have come up in our sexuality education classes over the years. We received thousands of letters from boys all over the world with new questions and experiences to share, and that's how this book came about.

This book is a companion to *The "What's Happening to My Body?" Book,* and covers many of the same topics, though not in as much detail. You don't need that book to use this one. The big difference between the two books is that this is an interactive book, with exercises, quizzes, and other activities that will help you learn about the changes that take place in your body during puberty.

This book owes a great deal to the many boys and girls who have been students in our classes over the years and to the families who have attended our puberty and sexuality workshops. Much of the material in this book was developed and refined with their help. Indeed, without their kind patience when exercises and activities didn't work out as planned and their enthusiasm when they did, this book would not have been written. We also owe a big thanks to the many men and boys who have written to us over the years, and to those who spoke with us personally while we wrote the book.

We hope you (and the friends and family members you'll recruit for some of the activities) enjoy the activities and exercises in the book and that it will answer some of the questions you'll have as you enter this new stage of your life.

LYNDA MADARAS
AND AREA MADARAS

1.

WHAT'S HAPPENING TO YOU?

Imagine that it's late on a dark, stormy night. All is quiet as you stare out your bedroom window into the darkness.

Suddenly, the storm clouds part. Moonlight floods your bedroom, striking your mirror. You turn to look at yourself and come face to face with the truth. There's no longer any doubt about it. Your body is definitely changing!

Perhaps the first change you noticed was the coarser, darker hair growing on your arms and legs and in places where it never grew before. By now, hair may even be growing on your face.

You may have noticed the whole shape of your body changing—broader, wider shoulders; thicker, more powerful muscles. You may be growing at an amazing rate. Your feet may seem too big and your arms too long.

Your forehead is becoming higher and your jaw longer and lower, so that it juts out more. Your body may have a new, unfamiliar odor. And you may be experiencing new and intense feelings and urges.

What's happening to you?

    A. You're turning into a werewolf.

    B. You're going through puberty.

B. Puberty Is the Answer

You're not turning into a werewolf; you're turning into a man! Puberty is the time in a boy's life when his body develops from a child's body into a man's body.

Luckily, puberty doesn't happen overnight, and it's nowhere near as scary as turning into a werewolf. Still, puberty does mean lots of change, and it helps to know ahead of time what to expect. That's where this book comes in. It explains how, when, and why your body changes.

But this is not just a book about puberty; it's also a book about you. It is filled with exercises, activities, and places to record what's happening to you. In fact, by the time you're through, this book will be not only *about* you, it will be *by* you as well!

HOW OLD?

The drawing below is adapted from a medical textbook and shows three boys in different stages of development. Can you guess each one's age? Write your guesses in the blank spaces below. The answer is in the box on page 4.

STAGES OF DEVELOPMENT

EARLY PUBERTY	MIDDLE PUBERTY	LATE PUBERTY
age _____	age _____	age _____

Adapted from J.M. Tanner, *Growth at Adolescence* (Oxford: Blackwell Scientific Publications, 1962). Used with permission.

PUBERTY CHANGES

- Hair is more oily; you may need to wash it more often.

- Skin is more oily; you may have problems with pimples.

- Nipples enlarge, darken in color, and may be tender or sore.

- Breasts may swell and may remain enlarged for a year or two.

- Sex organs grow and develop.

- Curly pubic hair grows on and around sex organs.

- Muscles are thicker and more developed, and body strength increases.

- Hair on legs increases and may darken in color.

- Feet enlarge and perspire more; foot odor may be a problem.

- You go through a growth spurt and your weight and height increase rapidly. You grow taller faster than ever before. Your feet grow first. Your arms and legs grow before the trunk of your body grows.

- Hair grows on upper lip and on cheeks.

- Shoulders are wider and broader.

- Underarm hair grows; you may notice more perspiration (sweat) and body odor.

- Hair may grow on chest, back, shoulders, or elsewhere.

- Hair on arms may increase and darken in color.

- Erections (when the penis gets stiff and hard for a while) happen more often.

- And during puberty, for the first time, a boy ejaculates—releases a teaspoon or so of a white, creamy fluid called semen from the opening in the tip of the penis. You'll learn all about ejaculation and these other changes as you do the exercises in this book.

Starting Lineup

Puberty changes don't happen all at once. First you notice one change, then another, then another. Often these changes happen in the order shown in the chart below; that is, first, the testicles and scrotum enlarge; second, pubic hairs appear; and so on down the list.

But things don't always happen in this exact order. You may find that the changes happen to you in a somewhat different order.

Use the chart below to keep a record of the order in which these changes happen to you. When you first notice one of the changes on the chart, put a 1 next to it. When you notice the second, put a 2 in the blank space next to that change, and so on, until you've filled in all the blank spaces in the *You* column of the chart.

If you've already noticed some of these changes, you can start filling out the chart now. (If you can't remember the exact order, just make your best guess.)

YOU	TYPICAL ORDER OF PUBERTY CHANGES
____	1. Testicles and scrotum grow larger
____	2. First pubic hair
____	3. Penis enlarges
____	4. Ejaculation (release of semen)
____	5. Height growth spurt
____	6. Shoulders broaden
____	7. Voice changes
____	8. Hair on upper lip or underarms

Your Life: Past, Present, future

Since this book is about you, let's look at your life. What's it like now? How is it different from the way it was in the past or will be in the future? Filling in the chart below will help you think about these questions.

	PAST	PRESENT	FUTURE
The way I spend most of my time			
The people I'm closest to			
My favorite thing to do			
The most important thing in my life			

GROWING UP

❝ It was great. I remember thinking, 'I'm not a kid anymore!' I loved it! ❞

—JOHN, AGE 26

❝ It took too long. I was a late bloomer. It was a relief when it finally happened. ❞

—MILES, AGE 21

❝ I was angry and embarrassed and scared. Nobody told me what was going on. ❞

—TERRY, AGE 18

❝ I was sort of confused because I didn't understand what was happening. It was kind of scary. ❞

—PAUL, AGE 34

❝ It was neat; it was cool. Sort of like 'the arrival.' ❞

—JOSEPH, AGE 20

❝ People make it sound like it's this big dramatic thing that all of a sudden happens one day. It's not like that. It's not like some guy pops up and says, 'Hey, kid, this is it. Now it's going to happen to you.' ❞

—JACKSON, AGE 33

❝ I don't really think about it. I just sorta go with the flow. ❞

—CHRISTIAN, AGE 9

❝ It's like one minute it was really cool and the next minute I was totally freaked out about it. ❞

—ZACK, AGE 17

What About YOU?

You've heard what these boys and men had to say; now it's your turn. On the next page, you'll find a racewriting exercise with space for you to write what you think. To find out how to racewrite, check out the instructions below.

✖✖✖✖✖✖ RACEWRITING ✖✖✖✖✖✖

Just write whatever comes into your head! It doesn't necessarily have to make sense, and you don't have to worry about spelling and punctuation. (Don't you wish your English class was this easy?) The key to racewriting is that you time yourself, and the only rule is that once you start writing, you can't stop until you reach the end of the page. Then check out how long it took you, and write the time in the watch at the bottom of the page.

If you get stuck, don't know how you feel, can't think of anything to say, write just that—"I'm stuck," or "I can't think of anything to say." Write it over and over again as long as you have to, just so long as you keep writing without stopping until you've filled all the blank space. Now no cheating by writing too big! The idea here is to get as many thoughts down as fast as you can. Good luck.

⚒ RACEWRITING ⚒

What are your feelings about growing up and the way your body is—or soon will be—changing? Are you excited, scared, or both? How far along are you? Do you wish you were further along? How do you feel about the changes you've noticed so far? Are you looking forward to the changes to come, or would you rather just forget the whole thing?

If you're already well into puberty, do you remember what you felt like before? Do you feel different now? What questions do you still have? What are you feeling right now?

Remember to write as fast as you can, and don't stop for anything! Get your watch ready so you can fill in your time at the end. Ready, set, GO!

_____

_____

_____

_____

_____

_____

_____

_____

_____

_____

_____

write your time here

Asking Questions ... Finding Answers

If you're like most boys, you probably have a lot of questions about puberty. Sometimes it's hard to ask questions about your body because people act like you should already know it all. But that's silly. No one "just knows" things; we learn from other people. So having questions is perfectly natural. We hope this book will answer some of these questions and help you learn the facts in a way that's fun and entertaining.

We won't pretend that this book will answer all your questions. For one thing, it's more an exercise book than a facts book. We have written a facts books about puberty; it and similar books are listed on pages 115–16.

No book, no matter how good, can answer all your questions. Fortunately, there is a solution close at hand. To find out what it is, solve the riddle in the box below.

RIDDLE

What's bigger than a breadbox, conveniently located right in your own home, and contains amazing amounts of information about the physical and emotional changes of puberty?

The answer to this riddle is at the top of the next page.

THE ANSWER:

Your Mom, Your Dad, or Whatever Adult(s) You Live With

These folks are the answer. They're the most logical ones to turn to when you have questions, need advice, or just want to talk about what's happening to you. They can understand what you're going through—after all, they've been through it too!

What if you're ready and willing, but your parents are too chicken to talk?

Or maybe you're the one who's all red in the face—too shy and embarrassed to talk.

If you've had these sorts of problems, you're not alone. Take a look at the next page.

ALL KINDS OF FAMILIES

You may live with one or both of your birth parents or with adoptive, foster, or stepparents. Or you may live with one or more grandparents, other relatives, family friends . . . you name it! There are all kinds of families. If the words we've used in the next few exercises (or elsewhere in this book) don't apply to your family living situation, just substitute ones that do.

> **❝** It'd be easier to talk to them if they were close to my age. **❞**
>
> —TOM, AGE 17

> **❝** I get a little embarrassed. **❞**
>
> —CHAD, AGE 17

> **❝** Parents don't want to talk about it. **❞**
>
> —PETER, AGE 13

> **❝** I wish they'd just bring it up first. **❞**
>
> —ADAM, AGE 14

> **❝** I'm afraid of asking stupid questions. People think I should know. **❞**
>
> —ANDY, AGE 12

> **❝** I feel like I need an interpreter! **❞**
>
> —GENE, AGE 14

> **❝** I wish they'd talk about when they grew up. **❞**
>
> —MICHAEL, AGE 11

> **❝** They've never brought it up, but I s'pose it'd be all right if we did talk. **❞**
>
> —JAMIE, AGE 10

Easier Said Than Done?

As the boys quoted above point out, talking to your parents isn't always the easiest thing in the world. If you have problems talking to your parents (or even if you don't), try the exercises on the next few pages. They'll help you bring up the subject and help your parents remember what it was like to go through puberty. They'll also help you get past the embarrassment that so often keeps parents and kids from talking about these things.

Remember When...

Explain to your parent(s) that you need their help with one of your workbook exercises. Then have them answer the questions below.

INTERVIEW I: When you were my age . . .

What was your favorite radio or TV show?_____

What kind of music did you listen to?_____

Who was your best friend?_____

What did you most enjoy doing?_____

What did you want to be when you grew up?_____

Where did you go to school?_____

Did they teach puberty or sex education in your school?_____

Did your parents talk to you about puberty and how babies are made?_____

Do you wish they'd talked to you more?_____

INTERVIEW II: When you were going through puberty . . .

Did you start to develop earlier, later, or about the same time as your friends?

_____

What were the first changes you noticed? How old were you?
How did you feel about these changes?_____

_____

_____

What did your parents tell you about puberty and how babies are made?

_____

_____

_____

erections shaving ejaculations pubic hair
wet dreams voice changes making decisions about sex
crushes using a deodorant dating perspiration
how babies are made

Talking About Puberty

In the conversation balloon above, we've listed some of the topics that parents and sons might talk about during the puberty years. Can you think of any others?

PART I

For the first part of the exercise, you and a parent will take turns filling in the empty balloon below. You go first.

In the balloon, write a puberty topic that parents and sons might want to discuss. Then pass the book to your parent and have him or her write one. Continue taking turns until you've either filled up the entire space (in which case you're both winners) or until one of you can't think of another topic (in which case the last person to make an entry is the winner). When you've finished, go on to the next page.

PART II

Look at the two conversation balloons on page 13 and pick the three topics that would be most embarrassing or hardest for you to discuss with your parent. Write the three topics in the spaces below.

☐ **1.** _____

☐ **2.** _____

☐ **3.** _____

Then cover up your answers, and have your parent list the three topics that she/he would find most embarrassing or hardest to discuss with you.

☐ **1.** _____

☐ **2.** _____

☐ **3.** _____

PART III

Now compare your lists, answering the questions and following the instructions below.

Do the same or similar topics appear on both of your lists? Put a checkmark in front of those items.

Other than the items that are the same on both lists, are there topics on the other person's list that you too would find difficult or embarrassing to discuss? If so, mark those items with checkmarks too.

Are there any topics on your lists that are so embarrassing they would be very difficult or impossible to discuss? Put a star in front of those items.

Almost all parents and sons have at least some degree of embarrassment about one topic or another, which can make it difficult to talk about these things. But by doing this exercise, you should have a clearer idea of just where you may run into difficulties. You may even find that simply doing this exercise and identifying the embarrassment have already made it easier to talk about these things!

Below are some other suggestions you may find useful. Read and discuss each suggestion, putting an "x" in front of those that might work for you.

_____ Have a third person (a doctor, nurse, or counselor) talk with both of you about the topic.

_____ Read books or pamphlets, or watch videos about the topic together and talk about it (see pages 115–16).

_____ Have your parent read a book or talk to another person and then share the information with you.

_____ Find another person (family member, nurse, doctor) to talk just to you.

2.
THE MALE
SEX ORGANS:
An Owner's Manual

The sex organs are also known as the *reproductive organs* because they are the parts of our bodies that make us able to reproduce—that is, to make babies. These organs are also called the *genital organs* or *genitals*. We have these organs on both the inside and the outside of our bodies. *External* means "outside." So you probably won't be surprised to learn that the sex organs on the outside of our bodies are called the *external sex organs*. They are also called the *external reproductive organs* or *external genital organs*.

In this section, you'll learn about the external male sex organs: the *penis* and *scrotum* (the pouch of skin that lies below and behind the penis). You'll also learn a bit about the *testicles,* two organs that lie within the scrotum.

By the time you've finished this chapter, you'll know what these organs look like, how they work, and how they change during puberty. You'll even be able to figure out how far along in puberty you are!

Circumcised or Not?

Circumcision is an operation in which the foreskin, a special skin covering the top of the penis, is removed. Today about 60% of male babies are circumcised in the U.S.

If you've been circumcised, you probably don't remember the operation because it's usually done when a baby is only a few days old. Older boys and grown men rarely have their penises circumcised.

Some parents (Jewish and Muslim parents, for instance) have their male babies circumcised for religious reasons. Some have it done because some, but not all, doctors recommend circumcision for medical reasons.

All boys—circumcised or not—should wash their genitals every day. During washing, uncircumcised boys should pull the foreskin back all the way or as far as it will comfortably go. The foreskin should never be forced to retract! If your foreskin isn't yet fully retractable, don't worry.

circumcised

uncircumcised

pulling back the foreskin

HAVE YOU BEEN CIRCUMCISED?

If you have been, your penis won't have a foreskin. If you're unsure, ask your parents. In fact, even if you are sure, you might ask them why they decided to (or not to) have you circumcised. If you were circumcised for religious reasons, you might ask when and where it was done, who was there, and how loudly you howled.

The Male Sex Organs

If you take a few moments to color in the different body parts, you'll remember them better. These are important parts of the body, so it's worth the effort. Just follow the instructions below.

P.S. The instructions call for a red and a blue pencil, but any two colors will do.

- Find the *shaft,* or *body,* of the penis and color it red.

- Next, find the *glans,* or *head,* of the penis and color it with red and blue stripes.

- The ring, or ridge, of tissue that circles the lower edge of the glans is called the *corona.** Color it blue.

- At the tip of the penis is the small *urinary opening,* through which urine (pee) leaves the body. Circle it in blue.

- Use your red pencil to shade in the coarse, curly *pubic hair.*

- Behind and below the penis is a pouch, or bag, of skin called the *scrotum* (or *scrotal sac*) that holds two egg-shaped organs called the *testicles.* You can't see testicles in this drawing, but find the scrotum and color it with red and blue polka dots.

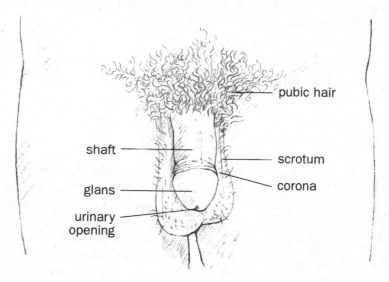

*Note that you can see the glans and the corona because this is a drawing of a circumcised penis. If it were a drawing of an uncircumcised penis, these parts would be covered by the foreskin.

Having an Erection

When the penis gets long and hard and sticks out from the body at an angle, you're having an erection. *Boner* is a slang word for an erection; when it's erect, the penis can feel so hard that it seems as if there really is a bone in there. But there isn't.

No Bones About It!

There are no bones inside the penis, just lots of soft, spongy tissue. During an erection, this spongy tissue fills with blood. The veins that carry blood to the penis dilate (open wider), increasing the blood flow. The spongy tissues swell up and become stiff with blood, which causes the penis to grow larger and become so stiff and hard that it rises up and sticks out from the body at an angle—and bingo, you've got an erection!

An erection can develop slowly or within a matter of a few seconds. Once erect, the penis can stay that way for some time, or the erection may disappear as quickly as it came. It all depends on the situation. Sooner or later, though, the veins constrict (become narrow) again. The extra blood that was in the penis is drawn back into the bloodstream, and the penis becomes soft and floppy again.

Men and boys and even little babies have erections. Often, they happen while you sleep, and one may still be there to greet you when you wake. You can have one when the penis is touched, when you're feeling "sexy" or having "sexy" thoughts, or when you're nervous or excited. Sometimes, especially during puberty, they happen for no particular reason.

Depending on where you are when it happens, having an erection for no reason at all can be kind of embarrassing. Check out the box on the next page to work on some ideas for how to cope with this if it happens to you.

During an erection the penis enlarges in size, becomes stiff and hard, and lifts up to stand out from the body at an angle. Some boys may also notice that the penis, especially the glans (head), deepens in color during an erection.

As the penis becomes erect, the scrotum becomes tighter, more rounded, and rises up, hugging the body more closely.

HOW DO YOU COPE?

Having an erection when you don't want to can be *sooooo* embarrassing. What are some things you can do to cope with this problem? Write your suggestions in the space below. Then turn the page and compare your advice to the advice we've heard from other guys.

_____

_____

_____

_____

What's Your Angle?

An erect penis may stick out at various angles, or it may stand nearly straight up. When erect, the penis may be straight or it may curve to the right, to the left, or some other way. No matter what your angle is, it's perfectly normal!

Erect penises may stick out at a variety of different angles

Shapes and Sizes

You may have seen pictures of penises (like the ones in this book) and been worried if yours doesn't look just like that. But penises can be many different shapes and sizes. Still, it's easy to get concerned if you're not sure what's normal and what's not. Here's the basic rule: Anything goes. Some penises are long; some are short. Some are fat, and some are skinny. And they're all perfectly normal!

Penises can be lots of different shapes, some of which are pictured at right.

The BIG Question: Is Mine Too Small?

Surveys show that most men either think their penises are too small or at least wish theirs were larger. In the letters we get from male readers, the most common questions and concerns are about penis size. So if you've worried or wondered about penis size, you're not alone. We hope the facts below will satisfy your curiosity and lay your worries to rest.

The Long and Short of It

For starters, you should know that the size of your penis has nothing to do with how macho, brave, or attractive you are. It has nothing to do with what kind of lover, husband, or father you'll be. Your penis size is a reflection of one and only one thing: the size of your penis.

About Average

There's a lot of disagreement among the experts about what's average. In general, though, the adult male penis is roughly 3 to 4 inches long when soft and roughly 5 or 6 inches long when erect. The shorter-when-soft ones grow more when they become erect, so they all end up being about the same size when erect. But don't get all flustered if your measurements don't match these numbers. For one thing, you're still growing. For another, you may not be measuring as far down the penis

---

TO COPE WITH ERECTIONS YOU COULD:

- wear baggy pants and long shirts if they keep happening
- shift your notebook to cover it or carry a book to hold in front of your erection
- sit down when you get an erection
- put your hands in your pockets to try and hide it
- tie a sweatshirt around your waist and let the sleeves cover it
- try to focus on something else until it goes away
- remember it's probably more noticeable to you than to anyone else

as they did. Besides, as you well know, your penis changes size, and not just during erections, either. Being afraid, cold, or nervous reduces the blood inside the penis, making it smaller in size. If you've ever waded into cold water, you know what we mean! Being relaxed or warm increases the blood in the penis, making it larger. And the stiffness and size of your erection also vary. So it's hard to say what the average size of one man's penis is, much less the average of all men.

Penis Enlargers

You've probably seen the ads. You know the ones—they try to make you feel like your penis isn't large enough just so you'll buy their product. Don't be taken in. These products aren't only stupid and pointless—they're also dangerous.

We've received countless letters from boys who have tried these products and were disappointed, to say the least. Basically, the kits contain weights you attach to the penis or scrotum. This doesn't really make the penis larger, but it can do permanent damage by stretching out the skin and tissue. In our opinion, calling these penis enlargers is S T R E T C H I N G the truth.

OWNER'S MANUAL

Routine Care and Maintenance of the Genitals

EQUIPMENT

- Washcloth and soap

MAINTENANCE SCHEDULE

- Clean at least once every 24 hours.
- On the uncircumcised model, the foreskin should be pulled back to ensure thorough cleaning.
- Apply clean underwear daily.
- For best results, do not use unclean athletic supporters, as this can lead to fungus buildup. (See "jock itch" in the Troubleshooting Guide on page 25.)

Injury Prevention

EQUIPMENT

- Jockstrap (athletic supporter)

PURPOSE

- To protect the testicles and penis while you're doing athletic activities.

TYPES

- Some fit like briefs; others are held on with straps (hence the name *jockstrap*).
- The soft-cup type holds the genitals snugly against the body so they don't get knocked around (though some guys feel that regular briefs do the job well enough).
- The hard-cup type provides extra protection for sports where you risk taking a hit to the groin. They are required by some schools and athletic programs.

SIZING

- Measure your waist! That's all you need to know to buy an athletic supporter, because the size has nothing to do with penis or testicle size. The cup will fit you no matter what size your genitals are, so all you need is your waist size.

- Adult sizes start in the 26-to-32-inch-waist range; youth sizes start at 20 inches.

BUYING

- If you know your waist size ahead of time, they're easy to buy. Just find your waist size and you're set! You don't even have to try it on!

- Jockstraps are sold in sporting goods stores and departments and in the first-aid aisle of some drugstores.

Medical Alert

SUDDEN, SEVERE TESTICLE PAIN

- **Following Accident or Other Injury:** Pain may be severe, but it usually does not require medical treatment.

  However, if pain doesn't begin to let up within an hour or so, if it worsens, or if there's bruising or swelling, see your doctor or go to an emergency room immediately.

- **Without Accident or Injury:** See your doctor or go to an emergency room immediately, even if the pain goes away as suddenly as it appeared.

Troubleshooting Guide

JOCK ITCH

- Dirty underwear or a sweaty jockstrap stuffed in a gym locker can be a breeding ground for a fungus infection that causes a scaly, itchy rash in the genital area. It can usually be treated with antifungals such as Tinactin, which can be purchased without a prescription. If the problem persists, see your doctor.

FORESKIN PROBLEMS

- The foreskin should never be forced to retract! If your foreskin isn't yet fully retractable, don't worry. But if it causes pain or discomfort, see your doctor.

Testicle Size

The drawing you see here shows an *orchidometer*, a string of wooden or plastic ovals of different size that doctors use to measure testicles. The numbers on the ovals of the orchidometer show their size in measurements called *milliliters (ml)*. By comparing your testicles to the ovals of the orchidometer, a doctor can make a good estimate of their size.

Measurements of testicle size are useful in determining whether or not a boy has started puberty, how far along he is in his development, how much further he has to go, and when he'll develop into a fully mature, adult male.

These measurements will also be used in some of the exercises in the following pages. The box below will tell you how to size your testicles.

SIZING YOUR TESTICLES

We couldn't include an actual orchidometer with this book, but we did manage to fit in the life-size drawing above that you can use as one.

First size one testicle and then the other (and don't worry if one is larger than the other; it's perfectly normal). You can size the testicle using one or both hands. You might want to hold the testicle up against the drawing, or you can stand in front of a mirror, book in one hand, testicle in the other. Do whatever helps you to decide which of the various ovals of the orchidometer is closest to your testicle in size. Then fill in the blank spaces below.

Today's date: _____ right testicle: _____ ml   left testicle: _____ ml

STAGES OF GROWTH AND DEVELOPMENT

One of the biggest changes in puberty is that your sex organs mature. Doctors have divided this process into the five stages described below.

Ages and Stages

In our descriptions, we give the average ages at which boys reach each stage. However, few people are exactly average, and there's a great deal of variation from boy to boy in when a particular stage will start and how long it will last. So we've given you not only the average age and average amount of time spent in each stage, but also a range of ages and times. That means we've given you the earliest and the latest ages at which boys are likely to start each stage, as well as the least amount of time and the most amount of time boys are likely to be in each stage. It's important to note, though, that these are just typical times and that some perfectly normal boys will start earlier or later than the ranges we've given.

Once you've read through these stages, try to figure out which stage you're closest to. Put a checkmark in the box next to that stage.

☐ THE CHILDHOOD STAGE (Stage 1)

This stage begins: when you're born and continues throughout childhood.
Starts: at birth.
Lasts: until puberty begins.
Testicles: are usually 1 to 3 ml in size.
Scrotum: increases somewhat in size, but there's no dramatic change.
Penis: increases somewhat in size, but there's no dramatic change.
Pubic hair: none.

☐ THE BEGINNING OF PUBERTY (Stage 2)

This stage begins: when your testicles start growing noticeably larger.
Starts: average is 10 to 12 years old; range is 9 to 15 years old.
Lasts: average is about 13 months; range is 5 to 26 months.
Testicles: have usually reached at least 4 ml in size and are at least 1 inch long. As development continues, one testicle hangs lower than the other (otherwise they'd knock together when you walk).

Scrotum: has also enlarged and hangs lower. The skin of the scrotum is thinner and not as smooth as it was in Stage 1. It's also reddish in color, though in dark-skinned boys this may appear as a deepening in color rather than redness.
Penis: may grow slightly larger, but basically there's little or no change.
Pubic hair: may appear in this stage or not until Stage 3 or later (see below). The first hairs are long and slightly curly and grow at the base of the penis and scrotum.

☐ THE LENGTHENING STAGE (Stage 3)

This stage begins: when your penis starts growing noticeably longer.
Starts: average is 12 to 13 years old; range is 10 to 15 years old.
Lasts: average is about 10 months; range is 2 to 19 months.

Testicles: continue to enlarge. They're usually 7 to 16 ml in this stage.
Scrotum: continues to develop as it did in Stage 2.
Penis: may have grown a bit wider, but the biggest increase is in length.
Pubic hair: usually makes its first appearance in this stage. It may be sparse at first. As development continues, it darkens, becomes curlier, and covers a wider area.

☐ THE WIDENING STAGE (Stage 4)

This stage begins: when your penis starts growing noticeably.

Starts: average is 13 to 15 years old; range is 11 to 17 years old.

Lasts: average is about 16 months; range is 5 to 30 months.

Testicles: are usually about 12 to 24 ml in size and about 1½ inches long.

Scrotum: continues developing as in earlier stages and skin darkens.

Penis: is a bit longer and quite a bit wider and the glans (head) is more distinct.

Pubic hair: has usually developed by the time a boy reaches this stage; however, as many as 15% of boys in this stage are without pubic hair. Once it has appeared, pubic hair continues to get curlier and eventually darkens in color and forms a triangle pattern. As development continues, it will spread beyond this triangle pattern and may grow up toward the belly, out onto the thighs, or elsewhere in the genital area.

☐ THE ADULT STAGE (Stage 5)

This stage begins: when your sex organs are fully developed.

Starts: average is 15 years old; range is 12 to 18 years old.

Lasts: the rest of your life.

Testicles: are fully developed at 16 to 27 ml in size and about 1¾ inches long.

Scrotum: is fully developed and deeper in color.

Penis: is fully developed and deeper in color.

Pubic hair: is fairly well developed but may continue to grow until about age 20.

The Growth and Development of My Favorite Person

Use these pages to keep a record of your development. Every 3 to 6 months, fill in another box. You might need to refer back to the descriptions of the different stages, which begin on page 27, or to page 26, which shows the orchidometer used to measure testicle size.

Date:_____ Puberty stage:_____ Testicle size (R):_____ml (L):_____ml

Changes I've noticed lately: _____

_____

_____

_____

Date:_____ Puberty stage:_____ Testicle size (R):_____ml (L):_____ml

Changes I've noticed lately: _____

_____

_____

_____

Date:_____ Puberty stage:_____ Testicle size (R):_____ml (L):_____ml

Changes I've noticed lately: _____

_____

_____

_____

Date:_____ Puberty stage:_____ Testicle size (R):_____ml (L):_____ml

Changes I've noticed lately: _____

_____

_____

_____

Date:_____ Puberty stage:_____ Testicle size (R):____ml (L):____ml

Changes I've noticed lately: _____

_____

_____

_____

Date:_____ Puberty stage:_____ Testicle size (R):____ml (L):____ml

Changes I've noticed lately: _____

_____

_____

_____

Date:_____ Puberty stage:_____ Testicle size (R):____ml (L):____ml

Changes I've noticed lately: _____

_____

_____

_____

Date:_____ Puberty stage:_____ Testicle size (R):____ml (L):____ml

Changes I've noticed lately: _____

_____

_____

_____

Date:_____ Puberty stage:_____ Testicle size (R):____ml (L):____ml

Changes I've noticed lately: _____

_____

_____

_____

Date:_____ Puberty stage:_____ Testicle size (R):____ml (L):____ml

Changes I've noticed lately: _____

_____

_____

How Much Longer?

Every boy is different, and no one can tell for sure how long it will take before you reach the adult stage, but the chart below will help you make a good guess.

Column I lists the stages, and Column II gives the average amount of time it takes to get from the beginning of that stage to the beginning of the next one. But few boys are exactly average, and the timing of these stages varies quite a bit. So Column III gives a range of times.

Example: Looking down Column I to Stage 3 and across to Column II, we see that the average time for Stage 3 is 10 months. Moving across to Column III, we learn that most boys will take somewhere between 2 and 19 months to get through Stage 3. (The other 6% will take more or less time than this.)

To estimate how long it will take you to get to Stage 5 and be finished with puberty, complete Parts I and II.

PART I

Step A. Find your current stage in Column I and read across the chart to Column II to find the average amount of time boys spend in this stage. Write the number of months in the square here.

Step B. Estimate how many months you've been in this stage. Write the number here.

Step C. Subtract the number in the circle from the one in the square. Write the answer here.

PART II

If you're currently in Stage 4 of development: Copy the number in the triangle into the star below.

If you're currently in Stage 3: Add 24 to the number in the triangle and write the total in the star below.

If you're currently in Stage 2: Add 34 to the number in the triangle and write the total in the star below.

This is the estimated number of months it will take you to reach Stage 5.

Remember: This is only an estimate based on averages; it may take you more or less time than this. But we promise you this: You will get there!

COLUMN I Stage	COLUMN II Average Time	COLUMN III Most Boys Will Take
2	About 13 months	5 to 26 months
3	About 10 months	2 to 19 months
4	About 16 months	5 to 30 months

TEST YOUR I.Q. WITH THIS P.Q.

(puberty quiz)

true   false

_____ _____ **1.** A boy who starts puberty at an early age will reach the adult stage sooner than a boy who starts to develop later.

_____ _____ **2.** If a guy finds loose pubic hairs on his sheets, pajamas, or underclothes, he should see a doctor.

_____ _____ **3.** Pubic hair is always the same color as the hair on your head.

_____ _____ **4.** If you haven't shown any signs of puberty by age 15, you should see a doctor.

_____ _____ **5.** Plucking your pubic hairs will keep them from growing.

_____ _____ **6.** The amount of pubic hair a man has depends on his racial, ethnic, and family background.

_____ _____ **7.** It's normal for the testicles to grow before the penis.

_____ _____ **8.** In earlier stages of puberty, the glans isn't as developed as it is in later stages.

_____ _____ **9.** Sometimes the testicles are closer to the body than at other times.

_____ _____ **10.** In adult males, the left testicle usually hangs lower than the right one.

TURN THE PAGE TO SEE HOW YOU DID.

ANSWERS

1. **False.** How early or late a boy starts to develop doesn't have anything to do with how fast he develops.

2. **False.** Just like the hair on your head, it's normal for pubic hairs to shed and be replaced by new hairs.

3. **False.** Pubic hair may be the same color as the hair on your head, or it may be lighter or darker. When you become an old man, your pubic hair may turn gray, just like the hair on your head.

4. **True.** There are many perfectly normal, healthy boys who don't go through puberty until they're 15 or older. But boys whose sex organs have not begun to develop by age 14 or 15 should see a doctor to make sure there isn't a problem.

5. **False.** If you pluck your pubic hairs, they'll just grow back. Besides, plucking these hairs hurts and could also cause an infection.

6. **True.** Men from certain racial and ethnic groups tend to have more pubic hair than men from other groups. A man's personal family background (what he inherits from his parents) determines how much pubic hair he has.

7. **True.** Testicles begin to grow at the start of puberty, and the penis usually starts to grow about a year later.

8. **True.** The glans becomes more noticeable in Stage 4.

9. **True.** When it's cold, the scrotum draws the testicles closer to the body to keep them warm. When it's warm, the scrotum hangs lower, allowing the testicles to cool off.

10. **True.** One testicle hangs lower than the other so you can walk without crunching them together. In 85 percent of men, it's the left testicle that hangs lower. But it's perfectly normal for the right one to hang lower instead.

There's Another Name for It

Use the space below to make a quick list of other names you've heard for the penis, scrotum, or testicles. Your list can include scientific or medical terms, baby words, and slang words, even so-called "dirty" words. (After all, this is your own private book.)

_____

_____

_____

_____

_____

You're No Dumb Elbow!

Chances are nobody's ever called you a dumb elbow, and we doubt that you've ever lost your temper and called someone a stupid foot. But take a look at the list you just made and think of all the names—both proper and improper ones—for the male sex organs. Then think of the insults and name-calling you've heard. We bet you've heard the names for the sexual parts of the body used as insults.

Why do you think people use sexual words to insult others? Use the space below to jot down your ideas about this. Then ask your friends and family the same question and compare their answers with yours.

_____

_____

_____

_____

_____

_____

_____

YOU SAID IT!

This will help you to pronounce words that may be new to you.

circumcised (SIR-kum-sized)
circumcision (sir-kum-SISH-un)
corona (kor-OH-nuh)
erection (ih-REK-shun)
genitals (JEN-uh-tuhls)
glans (GLANZ)
orchidometer (or-kih-DOM-uh-ter)

penis (PEE-niss)
puberty (PEW-bur-tee)
pubic (PEW-bik)
scrotum (SKROW-tum)
testes (TES-teez)
testicles (TES-tuh-kuhls)
urinary (YOUR-in-air-ee)

Puberty Disasters

Everybody has a puberty disaster story to tell. If it didn't happen to them, it happened to somebody they knew or to somebody who knew somebody they knew. Our friend Brian told us this one.

> In eighth grade, at the end of gym class one day, the big, macho football coach growls, "OKAY YOU GUYS, ALL OF YOU BRING IN YOUR NUT CUPS TOMORROW." So the next day, everybody shows up with their jockstraps. Except for one kid. He brings in his mama's nut dish, you know, her special nut dish she sets out when company comes. Needless to say, he never lived it down.

Trading Disasters

If you have a story better than our friend Brian's, use that. Otherwise, use Brian's story. What you're going to do is this: You're going to make a bet with your dad, your grandpa, big brother, or some other man in your life, someone you like or look up to.

You set the terms of the bet (loser pays for the popcorn at the movies, has to eat a can of dog food, give up his life savings—whatever). The bet is this: You tell him Brian's story, and he has a week to come up with a better one. If he does (be fair now), you lose. But you can take his story and go bet somebody else. Eventually, you're bound to win. When you do, write the winning disaster story in the space below.

_____

_____

_____

_____

_____

_____

_____

3.

THE INSIDE STORY

In Part 2, we talked about the external male sex organs—the ones on the outside of the body—and how they grow and develop during puberty. Before these changes on the outside of your body even begin to happen, other changes are already taking place on the inside.

Internal means "inside"; here in Part 3, we'll focus on the internal sex organs—the ones inside your body. Like the external sex organs, the internal sex organs grow and develop during puberty. In the following pages, you'll learn how these organs change during these years.

Both the internal and external sex organs are also known as the *reproductive organs,* and together they make up your *reproductive system. Re* means "to do again" and *produce* means "to make," so reproduce means "to make again."

You may be wondering "To make what again?" The answer is simple: It's you and me! Reproductive systems are what allow human beings to make more human beings—that is, to make babies. Of course, you're not ready to be a father yet, and won't be for some time, but during puberty your body is getting ready for the time in your life when you may decide to start a family.

What Happened on Your Birth Day?

Since we're talking about reproduction, let's talk about the day you were produced—your birth day! We don't mean the day you eat ice cream and cake and celebrate being another year older. That's your birthday. We're talking about your birth day—the day you were born!

Get ready to do an interview. Depending on your family situation, you might interview one or both of your natural, adoptive, or foster parents; your grandparents; or whatever adult(s) you live with. We've listed some sample questions. Adapt them to suit your family situation. For instance, if your adoptive parents weren't at your birth, you can ask about when they first saw you. And add some questions of your own.

Sample Questions

1. Where was I born? (city, hospital, etc.) At what time was I born?

2. Did I take a long time to come or was I born quickly?

3. What was the weather like on the day I was born?

4. Who else was there that day? (family, friends, medical persons, etc.)

5. How much did I weigh? How many inches long was I?

6. What did I look like?

7. How was my name chosen?

8. Did anything unusual or funny happen when I was born?

9. Can you tell me what else you remember about the day I was born?

The most interesting thing I learned about my birth day was:

_____

_____

_____

_____

_____

_____

_____

_____

_____

_____

Extra, Extra, Read All About It!

Now that you have an idea of what happened in your world on your birth day, what about the rest of the world? Your arrival was undoubtedly the biggest thing that happened to your parents that day. But you probably didn't make the front page of the paper. Who did? What was the headline story in the paper on your birth day?

A trip to the library will answer your question. Ask the librarian to help you find out the headline news on the day you were born. You can look at local, regional, and national newspapers in the library's collection of back issues. You might ask if *Time, Newsweek, Rolling Stone,* or any other magazine had an issue that came out the same day you did.

Make a birthday present for yourself. Photocopy one of the front pages or magazine covers published on your birth day and frame it!

Puberty Begins in the Brain

Long before you notice any of the changes of puberty, a part of your brain called the *pituitary gland* begins making increasing amounts of certain hormones. *Hormones* are chemicals made in one part of the body that travel through the bloodstream to other parts of the body to tell the body how to behave.

Your body produces all sorts of hormones. The pituitary alone produces so many hormones with such long names that we'd bore you to death if we tried to list them all. Instead, we'll just tell you that certain pituitary hormones travel through the bloodstream to the testicles, causing them to begin making a hormone of their own. This hormone is called *testosterone,* and it plays an important role in growth and development during puberty.

Sperm

During puberty, the testicles not only make increasing amounts of testosterone, they also produce sperm for the first time. *Sperm* are the male *seeds,* or reproductive cells. When one is joined with a female reproductive cell (called an *ovum*), a baby can grow.

Sperm are so tiny you'd need a microscope to see them, but they look something like tadpoles.

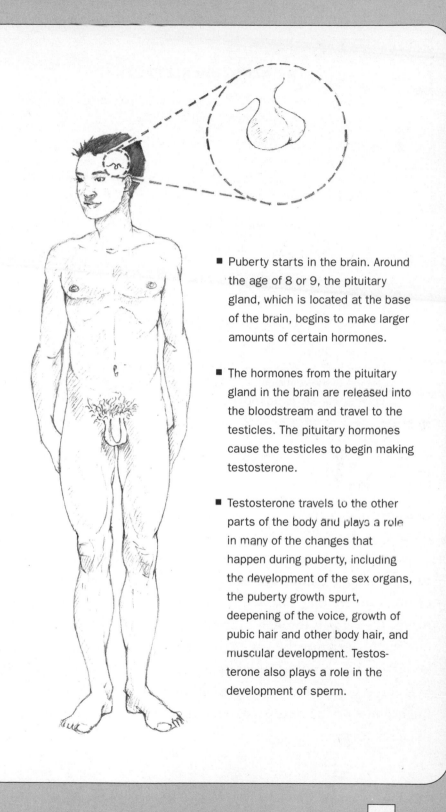

- Puberty starts in the brain. Around the age of 8 or 9, the pituitary gland, which is located at the base of the brain, begins to make larger amounts of certain hormones.

- The hormones from the pituitary gland in the brain are released into the bloodstream and travel to the testicles. The pituitary hormones cause the testicles to begin making testosterone.

- Testosterone travels to the other parts of the body and plays a role in many of the changes that happen during puberty, including the development of the sex organs, the puberty growth spurt, deepening of the voice, growth of pubic hair and other body hair, and muscular development. Testosterone also plays a role in the development of sperm.

AMAZING SPERM FACTS

- A boy begins making sperm in his testicles during puberty and continues to do so throughout most of his life.

- The testicles have to be just slightly cooler than normal body temperature to produce healthy sperm. So when it's cold outside, the scrotum pulls them closer to the body to keep them warm; when it's warm, the scrotum hangs lower so they stay cool.

- A normal ejaculation may contain 300 million sperm.

- If you laid 500 sperm in a line end to end, the line would only be 1 inch long.

- The average male makes about 10 to 30 billion sperm a month.

- You can't run out of sperm, and you can't use them up because your body is always making more.

- It takes about 2½ to 3 months from the time sperm start to develop in the testicles until they've passed through the epididymis and are ready to leave the body.

Ejaculation

During puberty a boy also ejaculates (releases sperm from his body) for the first time. Sperm begin to develop in the testicles and mature in coiled tubes attached to the top of each testicle. When a male is about to ejaculate, the mature sperm travel up into the body through a series of tubes, where they mix with various fluids. This mixture, known as *semen,* then travels through a tube in the center of the penis and spurts out the opening in the tip of the penis during ejaculation. In all, about 1 teaspoon or so of white, creamy semen is ejaculated. We'll talk about ejaculation in more detail in a bit. But first, try the coloring exercise on the next page to familiarize yourself with the internal male sex organs.

The Internal Reproductive Organs

Below is a simplified drawing of the male reproductive organs from the side view. If you take a few minutes to color in the various parts, you'll be able to remember what's what. These are important parts of the body, so it's worth the effort. Just follow the instructions below.

P.S. The instructions call for a red and a blue pencil, but any two colors will do.

A. Testicles. The place where sperm are made and testosterone is produced. Since this is a side view, you can see only one of the testicles. Color it red.

B. Epididymis. The long, coiled tubes attached to the upper rear portion of each testicle. Sperm mature here. Color the epididymis seen in this drawing with blue polka dots.

C. Sperm duct (or vas). The set of narrow tubes through which sperm travel as they move up into the body. Each vas runs from the epididymis (B), up into the body, and loops around the bladder (D). At the base of the bladder, it is joined by a tube from the seminal vesicle (F) and then enters the prostate (F), where it connects to the urethra (G). Color the vas shown in this side view blue.

D. Bladder. The place where urine (pee) is stored. It's not part of the reproductive system, but color it with blue stripes.

E. Seminal vesicles. The place where sticky fluid is made that is added to sperm and other fluids to make semen. Color the seminal vesicle seen in this side view with red stripes.

F. Prostate. A gland that adds more fluid to the semen. Color it with red polka dots.

G. Urethra. The hollow tube in the center of the penis. Both semen and urine leave the body through this tube (but never at the same time! See the box on page 47). Color the urethra red.

H. Urinary, or urethral, opening. The external opening at the end of the urethra, located in the center of the glans (head) of the penis. Circle it with blue.

Ejaculation: The Inside Story

Now that you have an idea of what the different parts of the internal reproductive system look like and how they connect to one another, let's look at what happens on the inside during ejaculation.

The drawing shows what happens shortly before and during ejaculation. As you can see, the penis is erect—that is, stiff and hard. (Remember we talked about erections in Part 2.) Not all erections end in ejaculations, but all ejaculations begin with an erection.

1. Shortly before ejaculation, muscles in the testicles, epididymides (the plural for epididymis), and sperm duct contract rhythmically, pumping sperm from the epididymides into the vas and up into the body (see arrows).

2. As the sperm reach this point, rhythmic muscle contractions squeeze fluid from the seminal vesicles into the mix. This mixture of sperm and seminal fluid is called semen.

3. More fluid is added to the semen here as similar contractions force fluid from the prostate into the mix.

4. Glands located here make a few drops of clear liquid called pre-ejaculatory fluid, which may appear at the tip of the penis sometime before ejaculation.

5. Actual ejaculation begins with powerful muscle contractions that propel the semen along the length of the urethra.

6. The semen spurts out the urethral opening in the center of the penis. It usually comes out in 5 or 6 spurts (though it may take more or less than this). On the average, 1 teaspoon of milky, white semen is ejaculated, but the amount varies from as little as 1/25 of a teaspoon to as much as 2 teaspoons. It spurts an average distance of 7 to 10 inches (if nothing is in the way). But sometimes, especially in young boys, it may only dribble out.

FINISH

START

Orgasm

When a male ejaculates, he usually has the intense, pleasurable feeling that is known as *orgasm*. It's difficult to explain exactly how an orgasm feels. Some people compare it to a sneeze because both involve convulsive spasms of muscle contractions. But having an orgasm is much more pleasurable than sneezing. Perhaps a better explanation is that an orgasm is an intense spasm or waves of pleasure that begin in the sex organs and radiate outward, sometimes involving the whole body. The intensity of an orgasm may vary from one ejaculation to the next, but most people agree that it's a pretty good feeling.

In addition to the changes described on the preceding pages, several other things happen before and during orgasm and ejaculation.

- The scrotum tightens, and muscle contractions pull the testicles closer to the body.

- The opening in the tip of the penis becomes more slit-like, and the head may become a deeper or more purplish-red color.

- The skin on the stomach, chest, neck, and face may get flushed or reddish in color. This is called the *sex flush,* and it happens in 1 out of every 4 males.

- The nipples may become erect and deeper in color.

- The heart rate and breathing will become more rapid.

- There may be muscle contractions in arms, legs, stomach, and/or feet.

- The body may sweat, especially the hands and feet.

After ejaculation and orgasm, the body returns to its normal state. This may happen fairly quickly or rather slowly. The penis becomes soft again and gradually returns to its normal size. Men usually feel relaxed and may feel sleepy after orgasm.

CAN YOU URINATE AND EJACULATE AT THE SAME TIME?

Because urine (pee) and semen both leave the body through the same tube, boys often wonder if it's possible for urine and semen to get mixed together. It's a logical question, but the answer is no. Urine and semen can't travel through the urethra at the same time. When a male is about to ejaculate, a special valve closes, preventing urine from leaving the bladder. So it's just not possible to ejaculate and urinate at the same time.

Some men are able to have another ejaculation and orgasm almost right away. Usually, though, there's a period of time that must pass—anywhere from a few minutes to a half hour, several hours, or a day or so—before a man is able to get another erection and is ready to have another orgasm.

First Ejaculation—When?

The age at which a boy has his first ejaculation varies quite a bit. The average age for the first ejaculation is around 13 to 14 years old. Nine out of ten boys (90% of boys) will have their first ejaculation between the ages of 11 and 15 years, but one out of every ten boys (10% of boys) will be older than age 15 or younger than age 11 when he first ejaculates.

First Ejaculation—How?

Most boys have their first ejaculation as a result of masturbation or having a wet dream.

WET DREAMS

About ⅓ of boys have their first ejaculation while they are asleep. This is called a *nocturnal emission,* or *wet dream.* Wet dreams can happen to older males, but they're more common among boys going through puberty.

It's called a wet dream because your bed or pajamas may be slightly wet from the semen ejaculated and many boys remember having a "sexy" dream when they awaken. However, other boys don't recall having a sexy dream, and some don't recall having a dream of any kind.

It's possible for a boy to have wet dreams without knowing it. He may not wake up right after the dream and there's really very little semen, so it may dry up, leaving only a slight water mark that may go unnoticed. But not all boys have wet dreams. It's normal if you do and normal if you don't.

The word *nocturnal* refers to nighttime. Actually, though, a wet dream could happen anytime you're asleep—if you took a nap during the day, for example. But you do have to be asleep. When you're awake, you might have a spontaneous erection (when the penis gets hard for no particular reason), but there's no such thing as spontaneous ejaculations, ones that happen for no reason at all. When you're awake, ejaculations happen for a reason, and during puberty the most common reason is that a boy is masturbating.

HARRY'S STORY IS YOUR STORY

Below is the beginning of a story about Harry's first wet dream. Harry's story is really your story because you decide what Harry does. Read the story and choose the response you like best. To continue the story, turn to the page indicated. In the box at the bottom of that page, you'll find more of Harry's story and more choices for you to make. Whatever you have Harry do is perfectly fine. There are no right or wrong answers. Just have Harry do what you'd do in the same situation.

Harry woke up one morning and realized he'd had his first wet dream. Harry felt:

a. proud. (Go to page 52.)
b. embarrassed. (Go to page 53.)

Masturbation

About ⅔ of boys have their first ejaculation while masturbating. *Masturbation* means "deliberate touching or stroking of the sex organs."

Masturbation doesn't always cause ejaculation. But once a male has begun making sperm, he'll usually ejaculate if he continues masturbating long enough.

People used to tell all sorts of stories about masturbation—like it'll make you go blind or grow hair on the palms of your hands, or even that you'd turn into a werewolf. None of these things is true. If they were, there would be a lot of hairy-palmed, blind werewolves on the planet because the fact of the matter is that most people masturbate at some point during their lives.

Questions About Masturbation

If you're like the boys in our classes, you probably have a lot of questions about masturbation. Use the space below to list your questions. Then compare your questions to the list of commonly asked questions that we've answered on the next two pages.

_____

_____

_____

_____

_____

_____

_____

_____

Commonly Asked Questions About Masturbation

1. Do most boys masturbate?

Yes, most boys (and men) masturbate. In fact, over 90% of men have masturbated to the point of orgasm at some time in their lives. Some start during puberty or younger, and others don't start until they're older. Still others never masturbate at all. It's normal if you do, and it's normal if you don't.

2. How often do boys masturbate?

Among those who do masturbate, the average 15-year-old male masturbates about twice a week. Some boys masturbate several times a day; some once or twice a day; some once or twice a week. Some boys masturbate less often than this, and some never masturbate.

3. What if you masturbate too much?

Unless it interferes with your normal activities (like going to school, doing homework or chores, or hanging out with friends and family), there really is no such thing as "too much." Your body sets its own limits. If it gets tired, you just won't be able to get an erection until your body has rested. If you masturbate a lot, you might find that your penis gets sore from all the rubbing, but it's not serious, and it'll be fine after you let it rest for a while. The fact is that masturbation isn't physically harmful in any way.

4. If you masturbate a lot, will you run out of sperm?

No, you can't run out of sperm. As we explained earlier, your body is constantly making millions of new sperm each day. There's just no way you could run out.

5. Is it normal to imagine things when you masturbate?

Sure. This is called *having a sexual fantasy,* and it's completely normal. Sometimes people fantasize about things they'd actually like to do; other times people fantasize about things that they'd be embarrassed or feel bad about if they actually did. Again, this is perfectly normal. Some people worry that their sexual fantasies are weird or that there's something wrong with them. But we can pretty much guarantee you that no matter what fantasy you've had, there are plenty of people who have had almost the exact same fantasy. However, if your fantasies are violent and you're worried about this, you should talk to a counselor.

6. Can masturbation affect your athletic performance?

There's really no evidence that masturbation helps or hurts your athletic ability. Some athletic coaches think it's a good idea for boys to masturbate before a big game because masturbation can be a good way of relieving tension and relaxing. Other coaches tell their teams not to masturbate because they think athletes perform better when they're a little tense. If you're an athlete, you pretty much have to decide for yourself.

7. Is masturbation sinful or morally wrong?

People have very different ideas about what's morally wrong and what isn't. Today, most people do not think masturbation is morally wrong or sinful, and personally, we go along with that point of view. In the past, many religions held that masturbation was a sin; and although many religious leaders no longer feel this way, some still do. But even if a religion's official point of view is that masturbation is morally wrong, that doesn't mean all the people in that religion, or even all the religious leaders in that religion, agree. It's sort of an individual thing, something you'll have to decide for yourself. If you're bothered by the idea that masturbation may be sinful or morally wrong, perhaps you should talk with your minister, priest, rabbi, or religious leader. Or perhaps you'll find one of the books listed on pages 115–16 helpful.

8. If you don't masturbate, what happens to all those sperm?

If sperm aren't ejaculated (like they are during masturbation or wet dreams), they are simply reabsorbed by the body.

9. How do I find out more about masturbation?

Okay, okay, we cheated here. This isn't really one of the most commonly asked questions, but we wanted to see what you had to say. Fill in your suggestions in the space below, and then turn the page to see what others have suggested.

_____

_____

_____

_____

_____

GETTING ANSWERS TO YOUR QUESTIONS

You could:

- look it up in a book
- talk to a doctor or nurse
- talk to your parents
- talk to an adult you know and trust
- talk to a teacher (especially a health or sex ed teacher)
- talk to a coach

YOU SAID IT!

Some of the words used in this section of the book may be new to you. The pronunciation guide below will help you to say these words correctly.

bladder (BLAD-dur)

deferens (DEFF-ih-renz)

ejaculate (ih-JACK-you-late)

ejaculation (ih-jack-you-LAY-shun)

ejaculatory (ih-JACK-you-luh-tor-ee)

emission (ih-MIH-shun)

epididymis (eh-pih-DIH-duh-miss)

hormones (HOR-moans)

masturbate (MASS-tur-bait)

masturbation (mass-tur-BAY-shun)

nocturnal (nock-TUR-nuhl)

orgasm (OR-gaz-um)

ovum (OH-vum)

pituitary (pih-TYOU-uh-tair-ee)

prostate (PRAH-state)

reproduction (re-pruh-DUCK-shun)

reproductive (re-pruh-DUCK-tiv)

semen (SEE-mun)

seminal (SEM-in-uhl)

testosterone (tes-TOSS-tuh-roan)

urethra (you-REE-thruh)

vas (VAZZ)

vesicles (VES-ih-kuhls)

HARRY'S STORY, CONTINUED

Harry was so proud that he:

a. told all or some of his family. (Go to page 54.)

b. felt very grown-up all day. (Go to page 53.)

Medical Q & A

The boys in our workshops and classes sometimes have questions about medical problems that affect the internal sex organs. On this page and the next, we've included some of these questions and their answers.

What would happen if a boy had only one testicle?

Most males are born with two testicles. Every once in a while, someone is born with only one or with an undescended testicle (see the next question). Or a testicle could be removed surgically due to disease, injury, or an accident that completely crushed the testicle.

Fortunately this sort of problem is not common. But even if this problem occurs, the reproductive system can still work normally. If a male loses one testicle, the remaining one can produce enough sperm, and he'll still be able to become a father. (Remember, a male makes millions of sperm each day.) A male's sex life is not affected by the loss of a testicle either. About the only difference a male would notice is that there's no testicle in the scrotal sac on the side of the missing testicle. Nowadays, doctors can put an implant made of a special material into the scrotum to make it look like there are two testicles.

HARRY'S STORY, CONTINUED

Harry noticed that his sheets were wet, so he:

a. let his parents know what happened. (Go to page 54.)
b. pretended to spill water on the sheets and changed them himself. (Go to page 58.)
c. just left it to dry because there was only a teaspoon or so of liquid anyway. (Go to page 60.)

What is an undescended testicle?

Before a boy is born, his testicles are up inside his body. Once he is born, they descend (come down) into his scrotal sac. Sometimes one or both testicles don't descend, and the boy has what doctors call an undescended testicle.

At times, cold weather, a cold bath, excitement, or extreme physical activity will cause one or both of a boy's testicles to retract, that is, to draw up close to his body for a while. But this is a temporary condition. It's not the same as an undescended testicle.

An undescended testicle is usually noticed when a male baby is born or early in life, and it sometimes corrects itself. Once in a while, the problem isn't noticed until puberty, in which case the boy must have an operation. This is done because there is a greater risk of cancer developing in a testicle still undescended by the time of puberty.

I was masturbating, and I didn't want to get semen all over my pajamas, so I put my finger over the tip of my penis just as I was ejaculating so nothing would come out. And nothing did, but for the last couple of days I've had this pain in my penis, and this milky stuff has come out. What should I do?

Retrograde ejaculation happens when the semen is prevented from spurting out through the opening in the glans of the penis during ejaculation. In older men, there are certain medical problems that can cause retrograde ejaculation. But in boys, it usually happens as it did for the boy who asked this question.

HARRY'S STORY, CONTINUED

Harry's family:

    a. was proud that he was growing up. (Go to page 60.)
    b. didn't make a big deal about it because they didn't want to embarrass him. (Go to page 60.)

Retrograde means "going backward." In retrograde ejaculation, the semen can't come out the end of the penis, so it's forced back down the tube in the center of the penis. It may be forced up into the bladder, which can cause the urine to be cloudy for some time. It's also possible for the semen to be forced into the prostate. Either way, there may be pain and a discharge from the penis.

In some cases, the symptoms may disappear by themselves, but if they don't, or if you have cloudy or milky urine or a discharge from the penis, see your doctor. You may have an infection in the prostate that needs antibiotics. (You may feel embarrassed telling the doctor, but you needn't be; doctors are used to these things.)

I have this lump in my testicle. It doesn't hurt. What is it? Is it cancer?

Though it's not common, it is possible for boys to get cancer of the testicles. When it does happen, a painless lump in the testicle can be the first symptom (see page 57 for other symptoms). But this doesn't mean that *all* lumps (or even most lumps) in the testicles are cancerous lumps. They aren't.

Many conditions can cause a painless lump in the genitals. Sometimes what feels like a lump is merely some part of the testicle— for instance, the cord that covers the vas deferens. Or the lump may actually be in the scrotum. Most of these are cysts—collections of fluid. Some cysts go away by themselves; others require an operation.

Most lumps are not cancer, but because some are, all lumps should be checked by a doctor. And you should also protect yourself by learning how to do TSE: testicular self-exam.

CHECK IT OUT!

Testicular Self-Exam (TSE)

What Is It?

Testicular self-examination (TSE) is a way of checking yourself for signs of testicular cancer. Teenagers and young men don't often get cancer, but when they do, it's likely to be testicular.

If caught early enough, testicular cancer can be completely cured. By doing TSE once a month, you have a better chance of discovering any cancer that develops while it's still in its early stages, when it's most curable. TSE takes only a few minutes a month, so it's definitely worth your time!

How Do I Do It?

It's easy! All you have to do is roll each testicle between your thumb and first three fingers until you've felt the whole surface (see Figure 1). It's a good idea to do it in the shower or bath because the warm water helps relax the scrotum.

Figure 1.

Remember, you're only checking the testicles, not the scrotum, epididymis, sperm tubes, or blood vessels that are also in this area (see Figure 2). Ask your doctor to show you the difference. The testicle should be egg-shaped, with a smooth surface and shape. Be on the lookout for:

Figure 2.

- **lumps**

- **irregularities in the shape or surface**

- **areas where the tissue is firmer or denser than the surrounding tissue**

- **pain in the testicle**

- **a dragging or heavy sensation**

If you find any of these things or anything you think might be abnormal, go to your doctor, clinic, or medical office right away.

How Often Should I Do It?

At least once a month. Pick a regular day for doing the exam each month—the day your birthday falls on, the first day of the month, the first Sunday, whatever helps you remember to do it regularly.

Be a Lifesaver!

TSE is really easy to do, but a lot of men don't do it simply because they don't know how. Now that you know how, why not pass on the information?

Give this book to your dad or some other adult male you care about and have him sign below once he's read about testicular self-exam.

TSE

I, _____, do hereby certify that I have read the page on Testicular Self-Examination and promise to do my best to remain healthy by practicing Testicular Self-Examination at least once a month.

_____
NAME

_____
DATE

HARRY'S STORY, CONTINUED

Harry doesn't usually change his own sheets, so when his parents asked him about it he:

a. told them he had a wet dream. (Go to page 54.)
b. just said he spilled a glass of water and left it at that. (Go to page 60.)

Invent Your Own Puberty Rite

Throughout much of human history, in culture after culture, a boy's entrance into manhood was marked by rituals, ceremonies, and customs known as puberty rites. Some of these puberty rites were pretty scary or dangerous—like the ones where a boy was sent out into the wilderness, unarmed and without food or water, to survive on his own for several weeks or more. When he came back—if he came back—he was considered a man.

Not all puberty rites were dangerous, though. Some involved feasting for several days and concluded with the boy sitting on a throne while everyone knelt down before him, laying presents at his feet.

Traces of puberty rites remain today in the bar mitzvah ceremony that Jewish boys go through following their thirteenth birthdays and the ceremonies still performed in some Native American tribes. But for the most part, modern boys have little or nothing to mark their coming of age.

We think it's time to bring back puberty rites (not the scary ones, the fun ones). You probably won't be able to sell your parents on the throne-and-gifts-at-your-feet routine, but why not invent a puberty rite of your own?

A modern puberty rite could take many forms: a special ceremony, a camping trip with your dad, a special gift to be passed on to the next generation. It could be anything—well, anything you can get your parents to agree to.

The first thing you have to do is decide when you'll have your puberty rite. You could pick a certain date (like a birthday), a particular accomplishment, or you could celebrate after some milestone in your growth and development. For example:

- **first signs of testicle growth**
- **first facial hair**
- **when your voice begins to change**
- **when your first pubic hair appears**

Any of these events would be a good choice, or think up some of your own. Pick the three you like best and write them here.

_____

_____

_____

Next, think about what kind of puberty rite you'd like. Use the space below to jot down how you might like to celebrate your transition into manhood.

_____

_____

_____

NOW TURN THE PAGE AND GET YOUR PARENTS IN ON THE PLANNING.

Note to Parents

Okay, parents, now it's your turn to get in on the act. We're inventing a puberty rite here, and we need your input to make your son's transition into manhood something special. First, we need an idea from you of what sort of event you'd like to use as a marker. You might choose a special birthday, or a specific pubertal change, like a changing voice, first facial hair or shave, first pubic hairs, first sign of testicle growth, or first ejaculation. Take a moment to write down three events you and your son might choose as a time for celebrating his puberty rite. You can use some of the events we've suggested, or come up with your own. Write your three choices here.

_____

_____

_____

Now think about the form this puberty rite might take. For example, you might have a special ceremony, go camping, or come up with a special family gift to be passed on to future generations. Write your ideas here.

_____

_____

Now all of you sit down together and compare your answers from this page and the previous one. Did you choose any of the same events? Of all the events you each came up with, which one do you think you'd like to celebrate? Write it on the first line below.

How do you want to celebrate this event? Were there any similarities in your suggestions? Now that you've seen each other's answers, talk about what you'd like to do, and outline your plans below.

_____

_____

HARRY'S STORY, CONCLUSION

Harry still had some questions about wet dreams, so he:

- **a. asked his parents.**
- **b. asked a teacher or school nurse.**
- **c. looked it up in a book (like the ones listed on pages 115–16).**

Adapted from *New Methods for Puberty Education, Grades 4–9*. Available from Planned Parenthood of Greater Northern New Jersey, www.ppgnnj.org/edu.

4.

ON YOUR MARK, GET SET, GROW!

Have you begun to grow out of your shoes long before they're worn out? Are the pants you bought at the beginning of the school year already up around your ankles? If so, it may be that you've started your puberty growth spurt.

The *puberty growth spurt* is a period of especially fast growth that rapidly changes a boy's size and shape. The growth spurt affects your bones, causing them to grow at a faster rate. One result is that your height increases more rapidly than when you were younger.

Not only do you grow taller faster, but you also gain weight more rapidly during the growth spurt. At the peak of the weight spurt, it's not unusual for a boy to put on 20 or more pounds in a single year!

This increase in weight is due in part to the fact that your bones get longer and thicker and therefore weigh more. Muscle development also accounts for part of the weight gain. (And by the way, along with this increase in muscle comes an increase in strength.)

Not only does your body get taller, heavier, and stronger, but the proportions of your body (the size of certain body parts in comparison with other body parts) also change. As a result, the general contour, or shape, of your body becomes more "manly."

Even your face is affected by the puberty growth spurt. In general, a boy's face becomes longer and narrower, and its proportions change, giving him a more adult look.

A boy's appearance changes a good deal during puberty. The information and exercises in this section are designed to help you understand how your size and shape change and help you adjust to your new look.

Growing Up and Up and Up: The Height Spurt

Height spurt is a term for the period of time during puberty when a boy's rate of growth speeds up for a while. For most of childhood, the average boy grows taller at a rate of about 2½ inches a year. In some boys, this growth rate slows down a little just before puberty begins, so that it's actually closer to 2 inches a year. But once puberty has started and the height spurt kicks in, the growth rate begins to speed up again. It continues to increase for a while until it reaches a peak. This period of fast growth lasts only a few months before the growth rate slows down again, dropping steadily until a boy has reached his adult height around age 20 to 21. This rise and fall in the rate of growth is clearly shown in the graph you see below.

THE HEIGHT SPURT

HEIGHT GAIN IN INCHES/YEAR

AGE IN YEARS

This graph shows how the "average" boy's rate of growth changes between the ages of 7 and 19. Notice how the rate slows, rises sharply, and then slows down again.

The graph is based on the average rate of growth in the so-called "average," or "typical," boy. But few of us are exactly average, and the height spurt is an individual kind of thing. When it starts, how long it lasts, and how much growth takes place can vary quite a bit from one boy to the next. No one can tell you *exactly* how the puberty growth spurt will affect you. We can, however, tell you what typically happens and give you a range of ages and inches that describes what happens to most boys. (Keep in mind, though, that some perfectly normal boys —about 5%—will fall outside these ranges.)

The Height Spurt at a Glance

When it starts:
Average—11¾ to 13 years old
Range—10½ to 16 years old

How long it lasts:
Average—2 to 2½ years
Range—1½ to 4 years

How much you grow:
Average—9 inches
Range—4 to 12 inches

Feet First

Actually, it's feet and hands first, because these are the first bones to be affected during the puberty growth spurt. Then the lower parts of the arms and legs begin their growth spurt, followed by the upper parts of these limbs. Then the spine begins to lengthen.

What does this mean to you? Well, it means that first you'll outgrow your shoes, then your pants, and finally your coats.

A Note About Measurements

Because we'll be talking a lot about height in this section, you should know how to read the abbreviations we've used here. When you see a single prime mark next to a number ('), that means the measurement is in *feet*. When you see a double prime mark ("), that means the measurement is in *inches*. So if you were to see 4'10", that would read "four feet ten inches." Get the idea?

Keeping Track

Since the height spurt is such an individual thing, why not make your own personal record of growth. Start now by filling in the first line on the chart on this page. Measure yourself every 3 to 6 months and jot down your height on the next line available in the chart.

YOUR GROWTH RECORD

Date:	Height:		Date:	Height:	
	feet	inches		feet	inches
	feet	inches		feet	inches
	feet	inches		feet	inches
	feet	inches		feet	inches
	feet	inches		feet	inches
	feet	inches		feet	inches
	feet	inches		feet	inches
	feet	inches		feet	inches
	feet	inches		feet	inches
	feet	inches		feet	inches

Taking the Measure of a Man

You won't be able to see changes unless you make accurate measurements. Since it's difficult to measure yourself accurately, we suggest you get one of your parents or someone else to help you.

It's best to measure yourself against a wall or doorframe with your heels, bottom, and shoulder blades pressed against the surface. Stand in the same place each time, so variations in the floor won't mess up your measurement. Measure yourself with your shoes off.

When you're being measured, look straight ahead. Have your helper check to make sure your chin is level and mark your height on the wall or doorframe. Then measure the distance to the floor using the same measuring instrument (tape measure, yardstick) each time.

How Tall Will I Be?

This is a big question for a lot of boys, and an easy answer is a tall order. We searched high and low for an answer, but there just isn't any easy way to know for certain how tall you'll be when you grow up. There are some clues, though, that can help you make a good "guesstimate" (a cross between a guess and an estimate).

WHO'S TALLER?

When James and Seth were 11 years old, James was 3 inches taller than Seth. Now that they're adults, who do you think is taller? The answer is in the box on the top of the next page.

Guesstimating

The three clues on the following pages will help you guesstimate your adult height. For Clue 1, you need to know your height at age 10. For Clue 2 you need your height at age 14. For Clue 3 you need to know your mother's and your father's present heights. (It has to be your birth mother and birth father; stepparents and adoptive parents won't do for this clue.) If you don't have the information needed for all three clues, just do the ones you can. If you're not yet 10, come back and do Clue 1 when you reach your tenth birthday. If you're not yet 14, come back to Clue 2 when you are. Note: If you have enough information to do two or more clues, don't be surprised if you come up with two different answers. (We told you these are only guesstimates.) One hint, though: Clue 1 will give you a more accurate guesstimate of your adult height than Clue 2.

CLUE 1

If you know your height on or around your tenth birthday, check out the special ruler on this page. The left-hand (shaded) side of the ruler is marked for a 10-year-old's height. The right-hand side of the ruler shows the corresponding adult heights. To estimate how tall you'll be when you're all grown, just follow these two simple steps:

STEP 1

Find your height at age 10 on the left-hand (shaded) side of the ruler and put a circle around it.

STEP 2

Now, staying on the same line as the height you circled in Step 1, look at the other side of the ruler. Put a square around the height you see there. That's your estimated adult height. For example, if you circled 4'6" in Step 1, then your estimated adult height is 5'9".

height at age 10	estimated adult height
5'2"	6'7½"
5'1"	6'6"
5'	6'5"
4'11"	6'3½"
4'10"	6'2"
4'9"	6'1"
4'8"	6'
4'7"	5'10½"
4'6"	5'9"
4'5"	5'8"
4'4"	5'6½"
4'3"	5'5"
4'2"	5'4"
4'1"	5'3"
4'	5'1½"
3'11"	5'
3'10"	4'11"
3'9"	4'9½"
3'8"	4'8½"

CLUE 2

If you know your height on or around your fourteenth birthday, this is the clue for you. On the special ruler on this page, the left-hand (shaded) side is marked for a 14-year-old's height. The right-hand side of the ruler shows the corresponding adult heights. To estimate how tall you'll be when you're all grown, just follow these two simple steps:

STEP 1

Find your height at age 14 on the left-hand (shaded) side of the ruler and put a circle around it.

STEP 2

Now, staying on the same line as the height you circled in Step 1, look at the other side of the ruler. Put a square around the height you see there. That's your estimated adult height.

For example, if you circled 5'4" in Step 1, your estimated adult height is 5'10".

height at age 14	estimated adult height
6'	6'6½"
5'11"	6'5½"
5'10"	6'4½"
5'9"	6'3½"
5'8"	6'2"
5'7"	6'1"
5'6"	6'
5'5"	5'11"
5'4"	5'10"
5'3"	5'9"
5'2"	5'7½"
5'1"	5'6½"
5'	5'5½"
4'11"	5'4½"
4'10"	5'3½"
4'9"	5'2"
4'8"	5'1"
4'7"	5'
4'6"	4'11"

CLUE 3

For this clue you'll need to know your mother's and father's present heights in inches. (Remember, birth parents only for this clue.) They'll probably give you their heights in feet and inches. You'll need to convert these measurements to inches. The special ruler on this page will help you do this. The left-hand (shaded) side of the ruler shows feet and inches; the right-hand side shows what these measurements are when converted to inches.

STEP 1

Mark your dad's height in feet and inches on the left-hand (shaded) side of the ruler. To convert his height to inches, just follow the line you marked across to the right-hand side of the ruler. The number you see there is your dad's height in inches. Write that number in the square below and in the square under Step 3 as well.

EXAMPLE: Owen's dad is 6'1" tall. Owen marks this on the ruler and sees that his dad's height in inches is 73 inches.

height in feet and inches	height in inches
6'6"	78"
6'5"	77"
6'4"	76"
6'3"	75"
6'2"	74"
6'1"	73"
6'	72"
5'11"	71"
5'10"	70"
5'9"	69"
5'8"	68"
5'7"	67"
5'6"	66"
5'5"	65"
5'4"	64"
5'3"	63"
5'2"	62"
5'1"	61"
5'0"	60"

STEP 2

Now do the same with your mom. Mark her height in feet and inches on the left-hand (shaded) side of the ruler. Staying on the same line you just marked, look at the right-hand side of the ruler. The number you see there is your mom's height in inches. Write that number in the circle below and in the circle under Step 3 as well.

EXAMPLE: Owen's mom is 5'6" tall. He marks her height on the ruler and sees that she is 66 inches.

STEP 3

Now add the number in the square to the number in the circle and write the answer in the triangle below and in the triangle under Step 4.

$$\square + \bigcirc = \triangle$$

EXAMPLE: Owen adds 73 to 66 and his answer is 139.

STEP 4

Divide the number in the triangle by 2. Write the answer in the diamond below and in the diamond under Step 5.

$$\triangle \div 2 = \Diamond$$

EXAMPLE: When Owen divides 139 by 2, he sees that the answer is 69½.

STEP 5

Now add 2½ inches to the number in the diamond. The result is your estimated adult height in inches.

$$\Diamond + 2½ = \underline{\qquad}$$

EXAMPLE: Owen adds 69½ inches to 2½ inches for a total of 72 inches. So Owen's estimated adult height is 72 inches.

STEP 6

Now use the ruler on page 69 to convert your answer from inches to feet and inches. Look at the right-hand side of the ruler to find the number closest to your estimated adult height in inches. Staying on the same line, look at the left-hand (shaded) side of the ruler. The number you see there is your estimated height as an adult in feet and inches.

Write your estimated adult height in the star:

EXAMPLE: Owen looks up 72 inches on the right side of the ruler and sees that this corresponds to 6 feet on the left side of the ruler. So Owen estimates that he will be 6 feet tall once he's finished growing.

MEDICAL UPDATE

GROWING PROBLEMS

Growing Pains. Muscle pains that come and go, most commonly in legs, thighs, and behind the knees, but sometimes in the arms, back, groin, shoulders, or ankles as well. The pains usually happen in late afternoon and evening. They affect 5-to-13-year-olds and in boys are most common in 13-year-olds.

The cause is unknown, but some experts believe the pains are due to strain produced because the bones are growing faster than the muscles.

If you have this type of pain, check it out with a doctor. Growing pains don't require medical treatment, but you should make sure that you're really having growing pains and not something more serious.

Treatment: Massages, a heating pad, and nonaspirin pain reliever.*

---

*Aspirin can cause serious problems for people under 15 years of age.

Osgood-Schlatter Disease. A fairly common problem that causes knee pain and swelling. It affects the upper portion of the shin (lower leg) bone, which is still fairly soft, as it doesn't fully harden until you're an adult. Rapid growth during puberty can cause muscles to pull and strain against the soft bone, causing pain and swelling around the knee. This condition is most often seen in boys around the age of 12 to 13. If you develop symptoms, see your doctor.

Treatment: Mild sufferers: For 2 to 4 weeks, lay off vigorous sports and exercises that stress the knee. Severe cases: The knee needs to rest for several months to a year. Very severe cases: A cast may be used to help the knee heal.

Scoliosis. Curving of the spine. It's most likely to occur during the growth spurt, but is more common in girls than in boys.

If it's not treated, the spine may curve permanently, limiting physical activity. The good news is that it's correctable, especially when caught early.

Symptoms: An S-shaped curve to the spine when you bend over, uneven shoulders or hips, shoulder blades that stick out more than normal.

Treatment: Mild cases: special exercises. Severe cases: a back brace for a time. Very severe cases: usually surgery.

The earlier it's diagnosed, the better. So get checked out by your doctor or school nurse on your next visit.

Slipped Capital Femoral Epiphysis. A rare condition in which the growing end of the thighbone (the femur) has slipped from its normal position. It's more common just before or during rapid growth and happens most often in boys between the ages of 11 and 13. About 70% of the people who develop this problem are overweight.

Symptoms: Pain in the knee, hip, thigh, and/or groin; a "click" in the hip; a leg that turns outward; in some cases, a limp.

If you have symptoms (especially if you have a limp), see a doctor right away. An operation is needed, and the earlier the better.

TEST YOUR   WITH THIS
I.Q.   P.Q.
(puberty quiz)

true   false

____   ____   **1.** As a general rule, boys who are on the short side throughout childhood will also be shorter than average when they reach their adult height.

____   ____   **2.** The growth spurt happens at different ages in different boys and is more noticeable in some boys than in others.

____   ____   **3.** Girls go through a growth spurt too, but theirs usually starts earlier than boys' and ends earlier.

____   ____   **4.** The average 11-year-old girl is taller than the average 11-year-old boy.

____   ____   **5.** The growth spurt affects the bones in your upper body and legs before it affects your feet.

____   ____   **6.** The legs start the growth spurt before the trunk (the part of your body between your neck and the top of your legs).

____   ____   **7.** The growth spurt usually starts around the time you reach Stage 3 of genital development.

____   ____   **8.** Most boys are in Stage 4 of development when they reach the peak of their height spurt and are growing at the fastest rate.

____   ____   **9.** Growth in height is usually fastest in the spring and summer.

TURN THE PAGE TO SEE HOW YOU DID.

ANSWERS

1. **True.** But it's not an unbroken rule. It is true that boys who are short in childhood are usually short as adults, but this is not always the case. Some boys start out shorter than their classmates but find that during puberty, they catch up or even surpass their classmates in height.

2. **True.** Boys may start their growth spurt as young as 10½ years of age or not until they're 16½, and there are some who start even earlier or later than this. A boy may grow a few inches, or he may grow several inches during his growth spurt.

3. **True.** Girls have growth spurts too, but the boys' growth spurt usually starts later and lasts longer than the girls'.

4. **True.** This is because the average girl starts her growth spurt two years before the average boy starts his. But eventually boys catch up and generally wind up being taller than girls.

5. **False.** It's the other way around—feet first.

6. **True.** But the trunk grows more.

7. **True.** The growth spurt usually starts around the same time that the penis begins to grow longer, which is the beginning of Stage 3 of development. This is usually about 1 year after testicle growth (Stage 2).

8. **True.** However, almost one-quarter (25%) of boys don't reach their top growth until they're in Stage 5.

9. **True.** This is true for all ages, not just puberty.

Are Grown-Ups Big Babies?

If growing up were simply a matter of getting bigger, adults would just be giant babies. Okay, maybe you know some grown-ups who act like big babies, but how many do you know who look like giant babies?

None, of course, because we don't simply enlarge as we grow. Some parts of the body grow more than others. This changes the proportions of our bodies (the size of certain parts of the body in comparison with others or with the body as a whole).

During puberty, the legs and the trunk of the body grow much more than the head, and our bodies begin to take on more adult proportions. In boys, there's also more growth in the shoulders than the hips, making the hips seem narrower in comparison and giving your body more "manly" proportions.

For example, in babies, the head accounts for about ¼ of the total length of the body and the legs for about ⅜. But the head doesn't grow nearly as much as the legs do, and by the time we're adults, our proportions have changed quite a bit. In adults, the head is only ⅛ of the total height, while the legs account for about ½ of our height.

| newborn | 2 years | 6 years | 12 years | adult |

To show how proportions change, we have drawn the male body at different ages as if they were equal in height. If our proportions didn't change, we'd wind up looking like giant babies!

Your Changing Face

The puberty growth spurt also affects the bones in your head and face. The head increases somewhat in size, but the more dramatic changes occur in the face. The face becomes longer, and its proportions change. The overall effect is that your face is narrower and less pudgy than it was when you were a little kid.

Some bones grow more than others. Although the entire face lengthens, the greatest increase is in the lower portion. One result is that your chin juts out more.

Your nose gets longer and wider and becomes more prominent. It reaches its adult size before the rest of your facial features. So if you feel as if your nose is too big for your face, it may be that the rest of your features just need a little time to catch up.

Your mouth also widens, and your lips become fuller. Your forehead is higher and wider, and the entire profile is straighter.

In some boys, these changes are quite dramatic; in others, they are less noticeable. Because you see yourself in the mirror each day, even dramatic changes may not be very obvious to you. The exercises on the next couple of pages will make you more aware of how facial features change during puberty.

These are photos of the same boy taken at different stages of puberty. As you can see, a boy's face changes quite a bit as he grows.

From J. M. Tanner, *Growth at Adolescence* (Oxford: Blackwell Scientific Publications, 1962). Used with permission.

Parental Pics

Get your parents to dig out some pictures of themselves when they were kids, before they went through puberty. Then get them to show you their high school yearbooks or maybe their wedding photos—any pictures taken after puberty. After you've had a good laugh over how they looked and what goofy clothes they wore, study their faces, noticing how they changed as they matured.

Face Matchups

Just to give you an idea of how much faces can change during puberty, we gathered together some "before-and-after-puberty" pictures. See if you can guess which kid turned into which adult by drawing a line connecting the pictures that go together.

The correct answers are printed upside down at the bottom of the page.

1.   2.   3.

A.   B.   C.

Answers: Number 1 grew up to be B; number 2 grew up to be C; number 3 grew up to be A.

PICTURE YOURSELF CHANGING

Paste in photos of yourself taken every six months or so. It'll be easier to see how much you've changed if you use the same camera and stand about the same distance from the camera for each picture. Photos from a coin-operated booth are great for showing the changes in your face. Or you might use photos that show your whole body.

Each time you add another photo to the page, write the date the picture was taken underneath it.

Weight Spurt

Not only do you grow taller faster during the puberty growth spurt, you also put on pounds at a faster rate. In fact, at the peak of the weight spurt (typically about age 14 or 15), it's not unusual for a boy to gain 20 pounds or more in a single year. The weight spurt lasts for 3 to 4 years, and most boys add 45 to 55 pounds during this time.

Part of this weight gain is due to the longer, thicker bones that you develop at puberty. But a large part of the weight gain is the result of muscle development.

Muscle Development and Strength

A boy's muscles also go through a growth spurt during puberty. Both the size and the number of muscle cells increase, so that the amount of muscle in a boy's body doubles during his muscle spurt.

Along with this muscle growth comes an increase in strength, but not right away. The muscle, weight, and height spurts all happen at about the same time. But the increase in strength trails behind by about a year.

Once strength does begin to increase, a boy's ability to lift, throw, hit, run, and jump improves. Because muscles in the shoulders, back, and chest are larger, the strength of arm pull and push (thrust) is increased. So is the strength of the hand grip. A boy's reaction time and muscle coordination improve as well.

This isn't simply a matter of having more muscles. The lungs and heart also grow larger and work more efficiently, which means greater endurance and quicker recovery from the effects of exercise.

Superman You Won't Be

If we're giving you the idea that puberty turns boys into hunks with masses of bulging muscles or enables them to leap tall buildings, we don't mean to. Each of us is different, and how our bodies develop is influenced by many things: what we eat, how much sleep and exercise we get, our general health, and our family background (what we've inherited from our parents and grandparents). How we develop is also a matter of basic body types. Turn the page to learn about yours.

What's Your Basic Body Type?

The three basic body types are shown here. Each of us has at least some characteristics of each type. Some people are almost purely one of the three and have hardly any characteristics of the other two types. Depending on their bodies, such people are said to be classic endomorphs, classic ectomorphs, or classic mesomorphs.

Other people have a more even balance of traits from each body type. But no one has a perfectly even balance, and every adult can be classified into one of the three basic types.

It's harder to classify young people because their bodies are changing so much, but see if you can identify your body type. Read the descriptions of each type, and put a checkmark next to the body type that is closest to yours.

☐ **Endomorphs tend to be round and stocky, with round heads, short, thick necks, more body fat, and short arms and legs. Classic endomorphs may start puberty early, but finish late.**

☐ **Ectomorphs tend to be thin and angular, with narrow bodies, little body fat, thin arms and legs, and long, stringy muscles. Classic ectomorphs tend to go through puberty late.**

☐ **Mesomorphs tend to be strongly built, with broad, muscular chest and shoulders, muscular arms and legs, and little body fat. Classic mesomorphs tend to go through puberty early.**

Many of the boys we talked to were not happy with the way their bodies looked and wanted to be thinner, heavier, or more muscular (or totally buff). Some said they wanted to change their bodies by dieting and bodybuilding.

It's true that dieting and exercise can change the shape of the body to some extent, but we each have a basic body type that doesn't change, no matter how much dieting and exercise we do. If you're the endomorphic type, it's important for you to know that you may be at a weight that is the perfectly healthy, ideal weight for you yet look heavier than your friends or classmates who are the same weight but are ectomorphs. By the same token, if you're an ectomorph, you may be slimmer than some of your friends, which is perfectly normal for you.

You should also know that dieting is not necessarily good at your age and that bodybuilding may not be the right type of exercise for people your age.

Exercising Right

There are basically three types of exercise: strength building (bodybuilding), stretching, and aerobic (endurance).

Bodybuilding

If your goal is to be totally buff and muscle-bound, you'll have to wait until you're mostly grown. Before puberty, it's pretty much impossible for a boy to develop big muscles because muscle growth is affected by hormones (the special body chemicals we discussed in Part 3). Before puberty, there just aren't enough of these hormones for you to develop big muscles. Lifting heavy weights before puberty isn't likely to produce the results you're looking for; in fact, it can hurt you because even if your muscles are strong enough to lift a heavy weight, your bones may not be. You won't snap in half, but you can do long-term damage to your bones.

The ends of your bones are still kind of soft while you're growing. They don't become completely hard until you've reached your full adult height. While these bone ends are soft, repeatedly lifting heavy weights can damage them and cause problems with your natural growth.

STEROIDS

Steroids are synthetic forms of the male hormone testosterone. Some people take these drugs because they can make the body build up muscles faster than is normal. But steroids are very dangerous, especially for teens, because they can interfere with your body's normal development. Besides, steroids work only while you're taking them. As soon as you stop, the muscles disappear. Steroids just aren't a good idea. If you really want to build muscles, you can get long-lasting and positive effects with proper exercise.

Some side effects of using steroids show up after only a few months:

Normal growth stops

Bad acne

Overly aggressive behavior

Testicles shrink

Breasts enlarge

Headaches, dizziness, nosebleeds

Others may show up months or years later:

Heart attack

Cancer

Baldness

Personality changes

Mental problems

Stretching

Stretching exercises help keep your body loose. When you stretch out a muscle, do so gently. Don't bounce up and down; instead, let gravity gently pull and stretch your muscles. Don't overdo it. If you want to stretch a certain part of your body, it's better to stretch a little each day than a lot all at once. Otherwise, you may pull a muscle.

Stretching exercises are mainly important before and after aerobic exercise. Stretching can warm up the muscles before aerobic exercise to make them looser, which decreases the chances of injury. Stretching afterward helps prevent stiffness.

Aerobics

This is the most important kind of exercise. Not only is it good for your muscles; it exercises your heart and lungs, too. Doing these kinds of exercises builds your endurance and helps keep you feeling good and fit.

Examples of aerobic exercises include anything that really gets your heart rate going, like running or walking fast. So if you're active in track or in team sports, you may be getting this kind of exercise already. But sitting on the bench doesn't count. You have to be actively exercising in order to get the benefits of aerobic exercise. Experts say you should do some sort of aerobic exercise for at least 20 minutes, three times a week.

Even if you're not into sports, even if you're a total klutz, you can still get the exercise you need. Take a brisk walk or ride a bike (but you have to actually pedal for the 20 minutes; no coasting). There are lots of things you can do to keep that heart rate up for the full 20 minutes.

Dieting

Dieting is a bad idea for people your age. Your body needs lots of energy to grow, and you don't want to risk denying it the nutrients and vitamins it needs. But even if you can't diet, you can eat smart! You should exercise regularly and make sure you're eating the right amounts of the right foods so your body has what it needs to grow.

Eating Right

A healthy diet is important, especially while you're growing. To stay healthy, you should eat reasonable amounts of a variety of foods. And no, we don't mean snack foods. You need to eat food from all five basic food groups each day. These are the five basic food groups.

Grains

This group includes bread, pasta, oatmeal, breakfast cereals, tortillas, grits, and all foods made from wheat, rice, oats, cornmeal, barley, or any other cereal grain. Whole grains, like whole-wheat flour, oatmeal, and brown rice, are especially good for you. Whole grains are high in fiber, iron, and B vitamins. Whole grains should make up at least half of the grain-group foods you eat.

Most foods in this group contain carbohydrates, which give you energy. Everyone needs carbohydrates to maintain their energy levels. But if you're trying to watch your weight, don't eat a lot more of these than your daily requirement. These foods can add weight if eaten a lot. This is especially true because we often eat them with spreads or sauces that contain a lot of fat (like putting cheese on your tortilla and making a quesadilla). On the other hand, if adding weight is your goal, this is the stuff for you!

Vegetables

This group includes all vegetables and 100% vegetable juices. Most foods in this group are important because they provide you with a lot of vitamins without a lot of fat or calories. However, beans, potatoes, sweet potatoes, and corn are also included in this group, and they can have lots of calories. Really high in calories is a baked potato that is piled with butter and sour cream.

Fruits

This group includes all fruits and 100% fruit juices. Foods in this group are especially important because they provide you with a lot of vitamins without a lot of fat or calories. Also, fruit can make a really good substitute for sugary snacks.

Milk

This group includes milk, yogurt, and cheese. Foods in this group are rich in calcium.

Some foods made from milk, like cream cheese, cream, and butter, have little or no calcium, and are not included in this group.

Meat and Beans

This group includes all types of meat, poultry, fish, dry beans, eggs, and nuts. Dry beans are also included in the vegetable group. All these foods are high in protein.

Being healthy means eating the daily requirement from each food group. To make sure you're getting a good mix and the right amount of each food group, you can find the right diet, *designed just for you*, on the Internet.

Get a Personalized Diet from the Internet!

What types and how much food should you eat? There's not one answer for everybody. It depends on your age and your level of activity. Find out what's right for you. Visit www.mypyramid.gov/kids. Find the list of subjects on the left side of the screen. Then go to "My Pyramid Plan." On the next screen enter your age, sex, and physical activity. Then hit "submit." The next screen tells you how much of each type of food you should eat.

5.

B.O. & ZITS: IS PUBERTY THE PITS?

No, puberty won't turn you into a smelly, pimply greaseball, though books, pamphlets, and videos for boys your age make it sound that way. You know the kind we mean—the ones that go on and on about "personal hygiene." They can make you feel really paranoid about B.O. (body odor), like you'll need to soak in a vat of deodorant every day. Or they make it seem that if you don't wash your face ten times a day and coat yourself with pimple cream, you'll be a permanent resident of Zit City.

On the one hand, puberty brings new body hair and the first facial hair, and some boys are excited about this. But it's also true that during puberty your perspiration (sweat) glands become more active, so you perspire more and develop an adult body odor. Oil glands in the skin of the scalp, face, feet, and elsewhere become more active too, and you may notice that the hair on your head is more oily or that you have more pimples.

Let's face it, you could probably live without these and some of the other changes in this chapter, but it's part of the package. Before you panic, read the information and try the activities and exercises in this section. They'll teach you the facts about these changes and how to cope with them.

Perspiration and Body Odor (Sweat and B.O.)

During puberty, your perspiration glands become more active, and your body chemistry changes so that you develop a more adult body odor. You perspire in the areas of your body that have more of these glands—under your arms, the palms of your hands, the bottoms of your feet, and the genitals. Perspiration is healthy, so let it pore! Washing your body daily and wearing clean clothes will help prevent body odor. Deodorant soaps can be particularly helpful. If odor or wetness is a problem, you can use an underarm deodorant to control odor or an antiperspirant to help control perspiration and cut down on wetness. These are available separately or combined in the same product. Baking soda can also be used under the arms to absorb wetness and odor. It's important to remember, though, that deodorants and powders are not substitutes for soap and water!

Foot Odor

If we all ran around barefoot, foot odor wouldn't be a problem. The gallon or so of perspiration our feet produce each week would simply evaporate into the air. But we wear shoes, which trap all that sweat close to our feet. This provides a warm, moist place for bacteria to grow. It's the bacteria that cause that rotten egg, sulfur scent on your feet and shoes. So what do you do? Here are some suggestions for taming the problem.

- **DON'T WEAR THE SAME SHOES EVERY DAY.** Shoes should have at least 24 hours to air out between wearings.

- **WEAR ABSORBENT SOCKS.** Natural fibers, like cotton, absorb moisture and allow air to circulate.

- **AVOID SHOES WITH SYNTHETIC MATERIALS.** Stick to natural materials like canvas or leather because they let more air in and out of the shoe. This keeps your feet cooler and dryer and makes them a less attractive home for bacteria.

- **POWDERS OR SPRAYS FOR THE FEET OR SHOES AND SPECIAL DEODORIZING SHOE INSERTS MAY HELP.** These products are available in most drugstores or pharmacies, but your best bet is to avoid letting the bacteria build up in the first place.

- **TOSS WASHABLE SHOES IN THE LAUNDRY.** This can help, but it may not solve your problem.

- **KEEP YOUR FEET CLEAN AND DRY.** Make sure that you dry them well, especially between the toes! Keeping the feet and shoes clean and dry is your best bet for fighting those smelly bacteria!

Pimples and Acne

Zits, whiteheads, blackheads—if they don't sound like a lot of fun, that's because they aren't. Unfortunately, they're very common during puberty; eight out of every ten teens develop pimples or severe forms of acne.

During puberty, oil glands beneath the surface of the skin grow larger and begin making more *sebum,* a white, oily substance that keeps the skin moist. The sebum can get backed up in the ducts of the enlarged oil glands and cause whiteheads or blackheads. Pimples can become infected, resulting in red, swollen, pus-filled ducts. The infection may break through the walls of the ducts, causing a more severe acne problem.

Many people have the mistaken idea that blackheads and other forms of acne are caused by tiny dirt particles beneath the skin and that washing your face several times a day will prevent these skin problems. Not true!

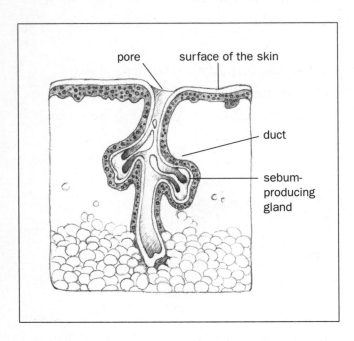

When sebum comes into contact with your skin's surface, it may turn black; it's this, not dirt, that causes the dark color of blackheads. Washing your face twice a day will help remove dirt and dead cells that would add to acne problems. But washing affects only the surface of your skin; acne is caused by what happens *under* the surface of your skin. You could wash your face a hundred times a day, but it wouldn't keep you from getting acne. In fact, washing too often may make the problem worse by irritating the skin and drying it out. This, in turn, causes the oil glands to produce even more sebum, which can lead to even more acne! And we hate to give you the bad news, guys, but males are much more likely to have acne problems than females.

So what's a guy to do? Fear not; there is help as close as your local drugstore. Check out the next page for information on how to deal with those little buggers if they show up. If you have a particularly severe case of acne and over-the-counter medications don't clear it up, don't just sit back and take it. Go see a skin doctor (called a *dermatologist*), who can help you. Don't suffer in silence; acne is a very treatable problem.

Acne Medications

There are a variety of acne treatments you can buy over-the-counter, without a doctor's prescription. Look for products that contain one of the following two acne-fighting ingredients.

BENZOYL PEROXIDE

The most common over-the-counter medication, it helps to fight acne by opening pores and killing the bacteria that cause the inflammation in a pimple. It makes skin feel tight and dry, but too much can be irritating to skin, so follow directions and don't overdo it.

SALICYLIC ACID

This medication is less irritating than benzoyl peroxide and even better at dealing with whiteheads or blackheads. So if this is your problem, this may be the stuff for you. Salicylic acid doesn't kill bacteria the way benzoyl peroxide does. Salicylic acid products can be used with other treatments.

If the over-the-counter products don't work, there are a number of effective medical treatments. See your doctor or a dermatologist for more information.

ACNE DO'S AND DON'TS

- **Don't** use oily sunscreens or lotions on problem areas. If you want to know if a skin product is okay to use, look for the word *noncomedogenic* on the label.

- **Do** wash your face regularly to avoid adding to an acne problem, but don't overwash or dry out the skin. Washing twice a day should suffice.

- **Don't** squeeze any form of acne, as this can make the problem worse and can even cause scars!

- **Do** keep a good mental attitude. Pimples are a drag, but they are perfectly normal. Try to keep a positive outlook and don't let those little buggers stop you from doing the things you want to do.

TEST YOUR I.Q. WITH THIS P.Q.

(puberty quiz)

true false

____ ____ **1.** If you have pimples during puberty, you'll probably have them all your life.

____ ____ **2.** Being nervous or excited can cause our perspiration and oil glands to become more active, which in turn may cause more perspiration and pimples.

____ ____ **3.** Boys are more apt to have pimples during puberty than girls.

____ ____ **4.** Blackheads are caused by little pieces of dirt under the skin.

____ ____ **5.** A good way of getting rid of pimples is to squeeze or pop them.

____ ____ **6.** Clean skin doesn't break out.

____ ____ **7.** There is no medical treatment for acne.

____ ____ **8.** Eating chocolate or greasy foods causes pimples and acne.

____ ____ **9.** Acne is often hereditary, meaning that it runs in families.

TURN THE PAGE TO SEE HOW YOU DID.

ANSWERS

1. **False.** Although some people have skin problems all their lives, most of us tend to outgrow our pimples by the time we reach our late teens or early twenties.

2. **True.** Nervousness, excitement, or stress can cause an increase in perspiration and pimples.

3. **True.** Boys usually have more trouble with pimples during puberty than girls do.

4. **False.** Blackheads happen because the oils that clog the skin's pores turn black when they come in contact with the oxygen in the air around us. Blackheads are not caused by dirt particles under the skin.

5. **False.** Squeezing a pimple pushes infected pus into the surrounding skin and can cause severe breakouts of acne and may result in permanent scarring. (African-American boys, be sure to read pages 107–8.)

6. **False.** Acne is the result of things happening under the skin's surface, so even clean skin can have acne.

7. **False.** Although acne isn't 100% curable, it can be treated successfully with over-the-counter medications or with the help of a skilled dermatologist (skin doctor).

8. **False.** Most doctors agree that eating chocolate or greasy foods does not increase your chances of getting acne. However, some people may be especially sensitive to certain foods, so if you notice that you tend to have more breakouts in the week following eating a certain type of food, try eliminating it from your diet and see what happens.

9. **True.** Acne does seem to run in families, so if your parents or older brothers and sisters had acne, you may be more likely to develop it.

Underarm and Other Body Hair

The word *puberty* comes from the Latin word *pubescere,* which means "to be covered with hair." Actually, most of the body is covered by fine, short, colorless villous hairs throughout childhood. During puberty, villous hairs are rapidly replaced by adult-type terminal hair, which may have some color to it. How much terminal hair you have, where it grows, and its color are determined by your racial, ethnic, and personal family background.

The curly pubic hair we talked about in Part 2 is a special type of terminal hair that grows on and around the sex organs. During puberty, villous hair in the armpits is also replaced by terminal hair. In addition, you may notice that the hair elsewhere on your body is darker in color, and that there's more of it.

Underarm Hair

Underarm hair usually doesn't begin to grow until a year or two after pubic hair growth begins. But this is not a hard-and-fast rule.

At first, underarm hairs are fine, straight, and only slightly colored. It takes about a year before more deeply colored, adult-type hairs appear.

Hair on the Arms and Legs

Early in puberty, slightly colored terminal hairs rapidly begin to replace the villous hairs on the arms. Terminal hair growth on the legs usually doesn't start until terminal hair growth on the arms is well under way. As we've said, the amount of hair and its color depend on your family background. Some boys have quite a bit; others have very little.

Other Body Hair

The hair growth on the upper legs may include the buttocks as well. In addition, some males grow hair on their chest, shoulders, and/or back. Others don't. Either way is perfectly normal.

Facial Hair

The first facial hairs usually appear between the ages of 14 and 16. However, some boys develop facial hair at a younger age, while others don't do so until they're 19 or 20 years old. The hairs usually appear during Stage 4 of development.

The first facial hairs are usually found on the outer corners of the upper lip. At first, they may be only slightly dark in color, and there won't be very many of them. But with time, the color will become deeper, and the mustache will gradually fill in, growing toward the middle of the upper lip. While the mustache is filling in, hair usually grows on the upper portion of the cheeks.

As you mature, your facial hair will get fuller and more deeply colored. Men who had hardly any hair at the age of 20 may have a full beard by age 30. Also, the facial hair may or may not be the same color as the hair on your head. It's a very individual thing.

Some men decide to grow beards and mustaches; others choose to shave their facial hair. Many boys feel very grown-up when they start shaving. You may or may not decide to shave; the choice is yours. If you think you might want to shave, take a look at "A Guy's Guide to Shaving," on the next few pages.

A GUY'S GUIDE TO SHAVING

Equipment

The first thing you need to decide is what type of razor you're going to use. Basically, you have two choices: a regular blade razor or an electric razor.

Blade vs. Electric

A blade razor gives a somewhat closer shave, but the big difference is in the "smoothness" of the shave. The blade razor cuts the hair at an angle, leaving only a slight tip of hair. The electric razor cuts nearly as close to the skin, but it lops off the hair straight across, the way a tree trunk is cut, and the cut feels rougher to the touch.

Also, blade razors give a clean shave. The blades scrape dead cells from the skin's surface, so that skin feels especially clean after blade-razor shaving. On the other hand, electric razors are more convenient and less likely to cause nicks and cuts. They also take less oil out of the skin and are a good choice if you have problems with dry or sensitive skin.

blade cut   electric razor cut

ELECTRIC RAZORS

There are two types of electric razor: rotaries and foils. They cost anywhere from about $30 to $100 or more, depending on the design and extra features (cordless, rechargeable, and so forth).

- **Rotary electric razors** have a series of tiny blades that fan out from a wheel and work on the same principle as a lawn mower. As you move the razor across your face, the whirling blades cut the whiskers.

- **Foil-type electric razors** have a thin piece of metal (the foil) that has hundreds of tiny holes in it. As you move the razor back and forth on your face, the whiskers poke through the holes and are sheared off by the cutting block that lies beneath the foil.

BLADE RAZORS

There are a number of choices here:

- **Disposable vs. reusable:** The big issue here is the environment. Disposable, or throwaway, razors just add to the mountains of trash we're leaving behind for future generations to deal with.

- **Multiple-blade razors:** The multiple-blade razor has two to five cutting edges. Single-blade razors have only one cutting edge. Multiple-blade razors give a closer shave, but they also scrape off more surface skin and are more likely to cause irritation (especially for those with sensitive skin). You're also more likely to get nicks and cuts using a multiple-blade razor.

- **Pivot and flexible heads:** Many multiple-blade razors have a cartridge that swivels and blades that ride on tiny springs to give you a closer, more comfortable shave.

  Men give these razors top marks according to an article in *Consumer Reports* magazine. But as the article also points out, shaving with one of these razors costs a little more.

Shaving How-To

How you shave depends on which type of razor you're using. But whatever razor you use, keep the following things in mind.

- **Take your time.** If you hurry, you are more likely to nick or cut yourself.

- **Rinse with cool water.** This will reduce irritation to the skin.

- **Don't share your razor or borrow someone else's.** Disease can be passed by sharing razors, so keep it to yourself!

Shaving with a Blade Razor

A man removes 15,000 to 30,000 whiskers when he shaves, and no matter how fine a razor he uses, this daily scraping can be rough on his skin. The following tips will help you avoid many of the skin problems caused by shaving.

- **Wetter is better.** The secret to a smooth, comfortable shave is softening the whiskers so they're easier to cut. The wiry hair shafts soften when they absorb water. By thoroughly wetting your whiskers before shaving, you can reduce the amount of force needed to cut the whiskers by as much as 70%. That's important because too much pressure and razor drag on the skin can cause *razor burn,* a red, stinging rash on the face.

  Some experts suggest shaving in the shower (using one of those fog-proof mirrors). Others recommend shaving just after you've showered. Still others advise wetting the face and applying shaving cream or gel and then letting it sit for 5 minutes before you begin to shave.

- **Use warm (not hot) water.** Warm water works best while you're shaving, but you don't want it too hot. Hot water plumps up the skin, so it's harder to get a close shave and easier to nick yourself. Don't forget to rinse with cool water.

- **Use a shaving cream, gel, or foam, not soap.** These shaving products help keep the hair and skin soft and reduce the drag of the razor across the skin. This reduces the chances of razor burn and infection. Don't use soap as a lubricant; it clogs the razor and dulls the blade. Besides, soap can dry and irritate the skin.

- **Use a sharp blade.** Dull blades drag across the skin more roughly and can cause irritation. Also, dull blades don't cut well, so you're tempted to press harder than you would with a sharp blade. Pressing hard increases the irritation to the skin. To make sure you're using sharp blades, you should change them after nine to eleven uses.

- **Shave in the direction of hair growth.** Shaving against the hair growth may give a closer shave, but it is much more irritating to the skin. For this reason, it's best to shave downward, in the direction of hair growth.

- **Save the chin and upper lip for last.** Your whiskers are thickest here; by saving these areas until last, you've given these whiskers that much more time to soften.

- **Rinse your razor after use, but don't wipe the blade.** Allow your razor to air-dry. Drying the razor with a towel or otherwise wiping the blade dulls it, shortening its life.

Shaving with an Electric Razor

- **Shave when your face is dry.** Electrics work best on stiff whiskers, so shave before you shower. You might want to use one of the shaving solutions made for use with electric razors, especially if you have a tough beard. These solutions are splashed on the face prior to shaving and are allowed to dry (which takes only about 15 seconds) before you begin to shave. They make the whiskers stiffer, which makes for a closer shave.

- **Don't press too hard.** Electric razors are supposed to glide across the face. Pressing harder won't give you a closer shave and could damage the razor heads.

- **Clean the razor regularly.** Some electrics come with a special brush or tool for cleaning; others simply have to be emptied out or rinsed under the tap. Follow the instructions that come with the razor.

- **Replace the blades each year.** Most manufacturers of foil and rotary electric razors recommend that the blades be replaced once a year. But here again, follow the instructions that come with your razor.

Nicks, Cuts, and Other Irritations

Everybody who shaves suffers minor cuts or nicks in the skin sooner or later. Since this is more likely to happen when you're new to the art of shaving, it's a good idea to have a *styptic pencil* handy to stop the bleeding.

A styptic pencil isn't really a pencil at all. It's a wooden stick coated with chemicals that help stop bleeding. You press it against the nick or cut and hold it there while the chemicals do their job. Styptic pencils are sold in drugstores.

If you don't have a styptic pencil handy, apply constant pressure with a clean tissue until the bleeding stops (usually within 3 to 5 minutes). Don't shave the area again until the cut has healed. If redness persists for more than a few days, see your doctor. If you find that you're cutting yourself all the time, switch to an electric razor.

RAZOR BURN

Razor burn is a red, itchy, irritated, inflamed condition that sometimes results from shaving with too dull a blade or pressing too hard while shaving. If you get it, you'll know because it hurts. Usually it goes away by itself, but if it doesn't go away after a few days, see your doctor, because it can become infected. Let the area heal before you shave there again.

RAZOR BUMPS

These can happen to anyone, but they are especially common in African-Americans and people with really curly hair. If you're African-American or have supercurly hair, read the information about razor bumps on page 107.

AMAZING SHAVING FACTS

Did you know that the average adult male . . .

- has between 15,000 and 30,000 whiskers on his face?
- has whiskers that grow an average of 0.38 millimeter a day?
- would have a beard 26½ feet long if he never shaved in his whole life?
- shaves 5 to 6 times a week?
- uses a disposable razor 9 to 11 times before he throws it away?
- spends about 3 minutes a day shaving? (That's 3,350 hours in his lifetime, or about 140 days!)

Ask a Man Who Knows

Your dad or another adult man you trust will have some helpful advice about shaving. Ask him the following questions:

1. How old were you when you started shaving?_____

2. What did you use to shave with the first time? Did someone show you how, or did you just pick it up on your own?

_____

_____

_____

_____

3. What type of razor and shaving products do you use now and why?

_____

_____

_____

4. Have you used other types of razors or shaving products in the past? If so, what did you use, how did you like them, and why did you stop using them?

_____

_____

_____

5. What advice do you have for me?

_____

_____

_____

_____

_____

░░░░ **RACEWRITING** ░░░░

You've gotten a lot of information about shaving! Do you have any thoughts about whether or not you'd like to shave? Why or why not? What helped you make your decision? If you decide that you do want to shave, what kind of razor do you think you'd like to try? Are you looking forward to the day when you grow facial hair, or do you think it sounds like a drag? If you've already grown some facial hair, how did you feel when you first noticed it? What questions do you still have? What are you feeling right now?

Remember to write as fast as you can, and don't stop for anything! Get your watch ready so you can fill in your time at the end. Ready, set, GO!

_____

_____

_____

_____

_____

_____

_____

_____

_____

_____

write your time here

Special Concerns for African-Americans

Acne treatments and shaving can pose special problems for African-Americans. Here's how and why and what you can do to avoid these problems.

Abrasive Soaps and Scrubs

Don't use them! They won't clear up your acne, and they may discolor dark complexions, causing patches of permanently lightened or darkened skin.

Razor Bumps

Because their hair is so strong and curly, African-Americans—especially those who shave—are more likely to have problems with irritation and bumps on the skin.

Shaving can make matters worse. Shaving puts tension on the skin and cuts the hair at an angle, leaving a sharp tip. Once the tension

Razor bumps: The tip of a curly hair can loop back, pierce the skin's surface, and grow inward. Shaving cuts hair to a sharp tip and increases the likelihood of this happening.

is relaxed, the hair can retract beneath the skin's surface, causing inflamed, irritated bumps on the surface of the skin. In some cases, these become infected and form large cysts, or collections of fluid, under the skin.

Shaving against the grain, with a multiple-blade razor, or with a dull razor can make the problem worse. Electric razors may help, but they are less effective than blade razors on curly hair.

The best way to avoid the problem is not to shave at all. If you don't want a beard or mustache, another solution is to cut the hair close to the skin with hair clippers, leaving a little stubble and a five-o'clock-shadow look. Some African-American men occasionally use chemical hair removers, but in order to remove the hair African-Americans may have to leave the chemicals on the skin for a long time, which means they have more chance to irritate the skin. If you use a chemical hair remover, *always* test a small patch of skin before using the cream. Use cream removers with moisturizers and natural herbs and oils (aloe, yarrow, rosemary, sage). Stay out of the sun, chlorine, and saltwater for 24 hours after applying these products.

Keloid Problems

African-American skin is more likely to form abnormal scars known as *keloids*. Scar tissue is formed as a part of the healing process when there's a cut, wound, or other damage to the skin. But in people subject to keloid problems, scar tissue continues to form even after the injury has healed, resulting in an extra build-up of tissue. The person is left with a raised, oddly shaped scar that may itch a lot. Even a little nick from shaving or popping a pimple can leave a noticeable scar in a person subject to keloids. Because of the risk of razor cuts and scarring from razor bumps, boys with keloids should consult their doctors before attempting to shave.

Voice Changes

During puberty, the larynx (voice box) grows larger and a boy's vocal cords become thicker and longer, changing the tone of his voice. A boy's voice deepens and begins to sound like a grown man's.

Girls' voices change too, though not as much as boys' voices. Male hormones cause boys' voice boxes and vocal cords to grow more than girls' do. In fact, males' vocal cords wind up being three times as long as females'.

Voice changes usually happen when a boy is about 14 or 15 years old, but it's perfectly normal for these changes to happen earlier or later than this. Your voice may change rather abruptly or it may happen without your really noticing it.

While their voices are changing, some boys experience voice "cracking." When a boy's voice "cracks" it suddenly shifts to a higher pitch, and temporarily sounds high and squeaky. Some of the boys and men we talked to say this was the most embarrassing thing that happened to them during adolescence. Others said it was no big deal. If your voice does crack, try not to worry about it. It's just another sign that you're growing up. You may also want to take a look at the quotes below to see what some other boys and men had to say about voice changes.

> **I think I was around 15. It was a real brief period where I'd get occasional cracks. You know, it didn't last more than maybe like a month, and from then on my voice just gradually got deeper, but it was a real gradual thing.**
>
> —CHRIS, AGE 25

> **If it cracked, it was no big deal. We all knew what it was, and it was happening to everybody.**
>
> —ADAM, AGE 17

Breast Changes

Over half of all males have some breast swelling during puberty, which may be accompanied by soreness and discomfort. The swelling may be more noticeable in some boys than in others. These breast changes are perfectly normal and rarely last more than a year to a year and a half.

There may be a flat, button-like bump under one or both nipples which may be sore or tender. Again, this is temporary. It's part of your body's adjusting to its new hormones and it's perfectly normal.

One change that is permanent is that the areola (the colored patch of skin around the nipple) gets wider and darker during puberty. This may or may not be very noticeable, but again, it's perfectly normal.

Some boys we talked to who have experienced these changes were a little worried. They thought that they might have cancer or something; one boy even said he was afraid he might be turning into a girl! He wasn't, of course. All of these changes are just a natural part of growing up.

Stretch Marks

With all the growing that happens during puberty, it's not surprising that some boys get stretch marks on their skin. On fair-skinned boys, they appear as purplish marks on the skin. In dark-skinned boys they may be lighter than the surrounding skin. Stretch marks usually fade with time.

Nearsightedness

Myopia is the medical term for nearsightedness. If you can see things up close just fine, but you have trouble seeing things at a distance, you may have myopia.

Myopia often gets worse during puberty and many new cases develop during this time.

Adam's Apple

Male hormones also cause changes in the angle of the portion of thyroid cartilage known as the Adam's apple. As a result, this part of the throat may become more noticeable.

Overwhelmed?

Have we overwhelmed you with puberty bummers? We didn't mean to. The changes described on these pages don't happen to everyone. We just wanted to make sure that if any of them do happen to you, you'll know what's going on and that it's perfectly normal.

Growing Up: What's In It For You?

Talking about things like B.O., zits, and other such bummers can make puberty sound like the pits. So we'd like you to remind yourself of all of the good things about growing up. Use the space below to make a list of good things about growing up—things you can do now that you're not a little kid anymore or that you'll be able to do once you're older. Then turn the page and see how your answers compare to those of other boys and girls your age.

_____

_____

_____

_____

_____

_____

IF YOU COULD . . .

Answer the following questions.

If you could be any age, what age would you be?_____

If you could be anybody in the whole world, who would you be?

_____

_____

If you could be anything you wanted to be, what would you choose to be?

_____

_____

Growing-Up Perks

Here are some favorites from other kids your age.

- More privileges
- Getting my braces off
- Getting a job
- Getting to stay out later
- Dating
- Being more my own boss
- Driving a car
- Getting into R-rated movies
- New friends
- Having my body get stronger
- Going to parties
- New school

- Having my own money
- More respect
- Joining the team in high school
- More allowance
- Making my own decisions (sometimes)
- Going to college
- Hanging out more with my friends
- Babysitting younger kids
- Getting really good at something (karate, art)

Picture Your Future

You've found a magic lamp, rubbed it, and out pops a genie who grants you a wish for the future. Complete the picture below by drawing a wish you have for your future.

FURTHER READING

Bell, Ruth. *Changing Bodies, Changing Lives: A Book for Teens on Sex and Relationships,* revised edition (New York: Times Books, 1998).

A fine book, representing many points of view through quotes from teenagers themselves. The section on teenage pregnancy is especially good, and the one on mental health, depression, and suicide is outstanding. The book is geared toward the 15-to-19 age group, but it could be valuable for younger and older people as well.

Calderone, Mary S., M.D., and Johnson, Eric W. *The Family Book About Sexuality* (New York: Harper & Row, 1990).

Designed for the whole family, this book talks about how sexuality begins when we are only tiny babies, and how it develops through puberty and adulthood, and even into old age.

Cole, Joanna. *Asking About Sex and Growing Up: A Question-and-Answer Book for Boys and Girls* (New York: HarperTrophy, 1988).

This was written for somewhat younger kids, but older readers will find that it answers many of their questions about puberty and sexuality.

Madaras, Lynda with Area. *The "What's Happening to My Body?" Book for Girls,* revised third edition (New York: Newmarket Press, 2007).

This is a book we wrote for girls about puberty. Needless to say, we think it's a pretty good one. Although it was written for girls, many boys and parents have read it and told us they learned a lot from it.

Madaras, Lynda with Area. *The "What's Happening to My Body?" Book for Boys,* revised third edition (New York: Newmarket Press, 2007).

This is the companion book to *My Body, My Self* in which we explain the body changes that take place during puberty. It has a lot more detailed information than we had room for in this book. If you have unanswered questions, we'd be willing to bet you'll find the answers here.

Planned Parenthood. *Kids Need to Know.*

This is an information kit for parents and teens that includes booklets and pamphlets on topics such as sexuality and birth control. The kit is available from the Information and Education Department, Planned Parenthood, 1316 Third Street Promenade, Suite B5, Santa Monica, California 90401.

Siegel, Peggy C. *Changes in You for Boys* (Richmond, Va.: Family Life Education Associates, 1991).

This book is short and concise (less than 50 pages), but it fully explains the changes of puberty.

Parenting/Childcare Books

Available wherever books are sold or directly from the publisher.

From Diapers to Dating: A Parent's Guide to Raising Sexually Healthy Children, *by Debra W. Haffner*

$16.95 (paperback) 978-1-55704-810-3

Beyond the Big Talk: A Parent's Guide to Raising Sexually Healthy Teens, *by Debra W. Haffner*

$16.95 (paperback) 978-1-55704-811-0

How to Help Your Child Overcome Your Divorce, *by Elissa P. Benedek, M.D., and Catherine F. Brown, M.Ed.*

$16.95 (paperback) 978-1-55704-461-7

Kids & Sports, *by Eric Small, M.D., F.A.A.P.*

$14.95 (paperback) 978-1-55704-532-4

Mommy, My Head Hurts: A Doctor's Guide to Your Child's Headaches, *by Sarah Cheyette, M.D.*

$12.95 (paperback) 978-1-55704-535-5
$22.95 (hardcover) 978-1-55704-471-6